REVIEWS AND PRAISES FOR THE STRATEGIES FOR MEN

This is a most fascinating report on the male dilemma. Personally, I think it is not just testosterone but attitude and behavior that set the stage for male deaths earlier. Anger is not a healthy mood!   Despite their stronger muscles, men have the worst mood of all-a dominance over and put down of women. We would not exist without the womb of a woman. It is tine to go back to the sane days of women as Goddesses

—C. Norman Shealy, M.D., Ph.D., Author of *Life Beyond 100*

* * *

Choosing the right parents prior to this current earth journey? Adjusting my diet based on my blood type and ayurvedic doshas? Fasting and praying? Morning Tibetan exercises or just holding my breath? Listening to the Elders? This and much more is Mr. Mamonov's fascinating attempt to live a long, healthy, and happy life.

—Velisar Rill, MD, Interventional cardiologists

* * *

I think it is very well researched and documented as all your books are. For the interested reader, certainly a treasure trove of new ideas and information. For some readers your "long excursion into the capillaries wonderland" could be a little deep, but as your book addresses the more than casual reader and the topic is very important I think you can keep it this way.

—Andreas Renfer, MBA

LONGEVITY MYSTERY SOLVED

THE STRATEGIES FOR MEN TO LIVE AS LONG AS WOMEN DO

VALERY MAMONOV, PH. D.

LONGEVITY MYSTERY SOLVED:

The Strategies for Men to Live as Long as Women Do

Valery Mamonov, Ph.D.

Amazon KDP Publishing

First Amazon KDP Publishing trade paperback edition January 2020

Cover design by Susan E. Smith

Manufactured in the United States of America

10 9 8 7 6 5 4 3 2 1

Mamonov, Valery, 1941–

Longevity Mystery Solved: Why Women Live and What Men Can Do to Extend Their Life / Valery Mamonov

pages cm

1. Healthy habits. 2. Heart and circulation.

3. Heart disease II. Title. [1. Self-help. 2.

Health. –Popular works.]

Includes references, glossary, and index.

RA776.75.M263 613'.0438 909-920

*This book
is dedicated to
my mother, Anna Danilovna,
guardian
throughout my life,
who continues
to guide me
from heaven
even still.*

CONTENTS

ACKNOWLEDGMENTS

Many people have helped me acquire healthy habits and become health-conscious which was not the case until I was 37. I am forever indebted to my Russian yoga teachers, Vladimir Samol and Eugene Bazh, from whom I learned various diets, exercises, meditation, body-cleansing methods, and the mind-body connection. They continue to guide me from the other side and I want to express to them my abundant gratitude.

I express my utmost gratitude to my editors, Norman Emanuel, Dr. Flora van Orden, Velisar Rill, MD, and Suzannah Sandler who spent endless hours painstakingly correcting my manuscript and making it readable and understandable.

Some of my research for this book is devoted to the heart disease and latitude connection from which I learned how deleterious to my health was living in the state of Maine for 20 years. Maine is reputed to be a "nice and cold" state. Although I lived in Russia in cold areas and used to a cold climate when I was younger, to me, Maine winters became increasingly cold as I grew older. In the depth of the winter, my hands would become frigid and circulation in them would be impaired. Eventually, I moved to Florida and I give my special thanks to my friends

Boris Klovsky, Valery and Jacob Barvashov, Walter Eizenberg, my daughter Victoria and her husband Stephen Mourousas and Kaori Yamane who aided me in my relocation.

I want also to thank my dear friends Vladimir and Slava Ostrov, who helped me to emigrate from Russia. They always encouraged me in my writings, provided me with their wise advice, and took my circumstances close to their hearts.

I would like to express my heartfelt thanks to Suzan E. Smith, for her guidance and expertise through the labyrinth process of publishing on Amazon and book cover design.

I apologize to any I have neglected to mention also worthy of my praise and thanks. This is not due to my lack of gratitude to them, but rather because of my failed memory.

INTRODUCTION

This book is an upgraded and modified version of Chapter 15 in my previous book, "Control for Life Extension. A Personalized Holistic Approach." While doing research for upgrading it, I became interested in some related health issues such as heart disease and cancer as related to food and they are discussed herein.

It is well established that in every country women live five to six years longer than men. Various factors such as smaller body size, higher body fat, lower hematocrit, renewal of red blood cells through periodic menstruation, and less hair on the body favor women's longevity. However, the most important factor is that men when they have sex lose their semen (life force) with the uncontrolled ejaculation, which women don't. Literally, sex kills men.

Men suffer twice as much from heart disease than women. Surprisingly, the latitude of the area where people live appears to be linked to heart disease. In general, the closer to the equator people live, the healthier they are and the less they suffer from heart disease. In cold climates, people burn food both for energy, necessary for all bodily functions and for heat to maintain their proper body temperature. In warm, particularly tropical climates people don't need to generate heat, they burn their food just for energy and avoid the production of metabolic waste, the byproduct of heat generation. Additionally, they sweat more and further rid their bodies of toxins and waste and this detoxification brings about better health.

To make their lives longer, men are advised to employ at least fourteen strategies including creating a healthy bank account, mastering the technique of controlled ejaculation (described in my book "Control for Life Extension"), avoiding iatrogenic (physician caused) disease, moving south or to higher altitudes, employing healing affirmations, being aware of a coronavirus egregore, and others.

Conventional treatments of heart disease such as bypass graft surgery or stent implantation to improve blood circulation are very invasive and drastic procedures. The heart itself is universally viewed as a pump with the ejection function only. Some opponents of this view stress that the suction function of the heart-pump must also be considered.

Furthermore, the shortcomings in the explanation of blood flow in the conventional cardiology text books are spelled out below. It is shown that the existence of the collateral blood vessels, capillary function (a second heart), muscle contractions (a third heart) and suction action of the heart's four chambers assisting the venous blood return must also be taken into account.

Dr. Ray Peat, a prominent American physiologist, once said, "Medical doctors don't understand human physiology." I feel that the same can be applied to conventional cardiology, namely that heart doctors and surgeons poorly understand how our heart and circulation functions.

Why are our foods so unhealthy and therapies so inhumanly invasive and drastic? The Concept of Gaia or Mother Earth helps us to find an answer to this difficult question. Humans exceedingly pollute and destroy nature and to protect Herself, Gaia punishes them making them sick and mass murdering them. It seems, Her envoys such as dictators and mass killers responsible for millions of deaths are granted a long life. It may sound as farfetched but maybe there is something to it.

1

1

WHY WOMEN LIVE LONGER THAN MEN

Each of us, man or woman, owes to our mother, a woman, the fact that we walk on the surface of Earth. In the process of our delivery, our mothers suffered excruciating pain and experienced loads of discomfort later on while bringing us up. For all this travail and effort that they endured, women deserve the best that life can offer–a long and happy life. In every country of this planet women live longer than men: we know in our hearts that it ought to be this way.

For decades, researchers were trying to find out the reasons why women live longer. Although they did not find yet a definite answer, they offered some inferences. "We know that biological, behavioral, and environmental factors all contribute to the fact that women live longer than men; but we don't know exactly how strong the relative contribution of each of these factors is" [1].

As far as long life is concerned, there is no doubt that women are superior to men. Jeanne Calment of France, world absolute champion of longevity, who lived to the age of 122 years, was a woman [2]. Among 50 supercentenarians (110 years and older) interviewed and photographed by Jerry Friedman in 13 countries, 40 or 80% were women [3].

In the Tokyo Centenarian Study of an outstanding number of 269 centenarians, women comprised a high 75% [4]. The percentage of women centenarians in the New England Centenarian Study in the USA was as high as 85% [5]. Among 11,048 people who reached the centenary mark between 1995 and 2013 in the UK, 81% were women [6]. In a study of 165 Italian centenarians, women represented 118 or 71.5% [7].

Across the world, life expectancy is much higher in the affluent countries (85-90 years) than in the developing countries (40-50 years in Africa). The gap between the life span of men and women is 3 to 4 years in the USA, Canada, and Western Europe, but increasing to 7-8 years in Eastern Europe (Poland, Romania) and further increasing to 10-12 years in transition countries (Lithuania, Belarus) [8]. In Russia, men have 13 years shorter lives. Over-smoking and over-drinking dramatically shorten the life spans of men in these countries [6].

We can consider a few reasons why women live longer. The hematocrit (volume occupied by red blood cells in the blood) in women is on the average lower in women than men, 42% and 47% respectively [9, p.1035], which increases the thickness of men's blood. Thick blood is to our detriment because thick blood kills [10].

The next life-shortening feature of men is that they do not menstruate. This inborn "defect" badly affects the quality of their red blood cells. The lifespan of red blood cells is about 120 days and before dying they lose elasticity, become rigid, and less than functional impairing blood flow in the capillaries. Premenopausal women menstruate at least four times within the span of a few decades and generate new deformable blood cells in place of those lost. This improves their microcirculation and spares them from thrombi formation.

Then comes a big one, namely when women are making love, they do not lose the essence of their life force as men do losing semen with uncontrolled ejaculation. Men, especially elderly folks, are warned to not overindulge in sex, otherwise, they can experience a "Raphael death." Raphael Santi, a famous Italian artist died at the age of 37 because he could not stop making love to his girlfriend, as historical rumors go [11]. Men can master a special technique described in the Sex Control chapter of my book [12].

As if it were not bad enough, women are also smaller than men in size and in every species across the animal kingdom individuals with a smaller stature enjoy greater longevity [13]. Besides, women have a higher percentage of body fat, 25% versus 15% in men which gives them extra protection in case of wasting diseases and a better adaptation to cold [14].

An unexpected longevity advantage comes from the fact that women are more naked than men. Among both animals and humans, the naked mole rats have the highest Longevity Quotient (LQ) of all living creatures [15, p.12] and women come next. The point is that women do not grow hair on their faces, thus avoiding a substantial loss of life force and energy that is otherwise spent on hair protein synthesis. Instead, they use their superior ability to synthesize proteins and fats by growing a child inside their bodies.

While pregnant, a woman's body produces Human Chorionic Gonadotropin (HCG), Progesterone, Prolactin, Estrogen, and Oxytocin hormones, and injections of urine of pregnant women were allegedly used in Russia as a rejuvenating medicine [16].

As mentioned above, in pregnant women the placenta produces HCG hormone, and urine of pregnant women is regarded as a promising medicine for penile growth in people with micro-penis. Women find it difficult to be satisfied if their vagina finds a tiny something jerking inside of it, therefore women took affairs into their own hands and started to produce HCG hormone for a penis to grow, you know.

The study found that testosterone was elevated and, "Mean penile length also increased significantly 24 weeks after treatment (flaccid length: from 3.39±1.03 cm to 5.14±1.39 cm; stretched length: from 5.41±1.43 cm to 7.45±1.70 cm; p<0.001)" [17]. Although not indicated in the study, the penis probably enlarged in thickness, too. Because some vaginas like it larger in all dimensions.

Twice upon a time, back in Moscow, Russia, I was standing on the subway escalator going up when a drunken woman approached me and asked if I had a thick one. I said no, and she expressed disappointment on her face. One of my former colleagues allegedly had one and after the date with his fiancée, she ended up in the emergency room bleeding. He was a real gentleman, and he married her.

As with many other things, we need to practice moderation (motto of centenarians) dealing with the HCG hormone. Overindulgence can be unhealthy as in the case of Kevin Trudeau who recommended it for overweight people and now serves a term in jail for allegedly unsupported claims in his weight loss book. So, moderation is the key, both with the HCG hormone itself and the consequences of its applications.

2
____

WHAT MEN CAN DO TO EXTEND THEIR LIFE

Age is an issue of mind over matter. If you don't mind, it doesn't matter.
— Mark Twain

Men can learn a great deal from women, centenarians and long living animals as well. To achieve longer life, their strategies may include but not limited to the following ventures (or adventures if you prefer):

1. *Know your body and personality type*. We are all unique. Thou shalt know thyself. Do self-assessment. My book [12] helps you understand your unique body and personality type and do everything right for your type. Eight Western and five Oriental diagnostic systems are used for self-assessment: heredity, lifestyle, Blood type, metabolic type, somatotype, personality type, instincts, temperaments, Ayurvedic dosha type, Yin-Yang type, Five Elements type, Chakra profile, and personal horoscope. Self-assessment is done through charts-you highlight entries in the charts that are appropriate for you, count them and put result of the assessment on the graph. After you are done through all 13 systems, you will have your unique multifaceted profile. Food choices for your type are at the end of that book. Other features of lifestyle suitable to your type are dispersed throughout the book.

2. Create a "healthy bank balance" by dramatically increasing your income. Although in England women live longer as in other high-income countries, in some districts of London, such as Belgravia, Kensington and Chelsea, men live longer than women [18]. In a study of 2501 elderly people in the USA, an annual income of less than $50,000 was found to be a risk factor for increased mortality [19]. Harvard Health Publishing in the July 2010 issue stated that, "Many men marry for love, some for money, and others for a variety of personal and family reasons." It also reported that unmarried men are at 82% higher risk of dying from heart disease than married men. Single men are advised to make "wise choices about diet, exercise, alcohol, and other health behaviors" [20].

The fastest way to jump to your new status is to marry for money. "Love and marriage, love and marriage, Go together like a horse and carriage," forget this outdated stuff. A few months later, after a few too many fights with your wife who doesn't comply, you will find your heart palpitating like that of an overdriven horse and spend the remnants of your money on divorce expenses with your carriage. **Marriage for love-No, marriage for money-Yes!** Men should go on a cruise ship, find a rich woman and marry her. To start your hunt, just ask how many cruises woman did. If it is in excess of fifty, then she is probably rich. Together with being very wealthy, a woman must be less than attractive. Then, you perform your marital duties rarely, if at all, preserve your life essence and prolong your life.

3. Learn how to control your ejaculation while making love. This is a critical skill; don't take it lightly.

In the animal model, both worker and soldier males in the naked mole rats community of 75 on average and living in burrows in the African Kenya, Somalia and Ethiopia, are not allowed access to the body of their queen, the only female producing offspring, except for a few selected ones. Among other factors such as breathing air depleted of oxygen, naked mole rats live 30 years as compared to 2.5 years of mice of the same body size which are not restricted in their sexual activities.

In humans, a good example is "…eunuchs whose testicles had been removed before puberty." The historical records of the Imperial Court of the Chosun Dynasty in Korea in the 19th century revealed that, "… the eunuchs lived for around 70 years–compared to an average of just 50 years among the other men in the court" [21].

In the United States, a cohort of 10,026 Roman Catholic priests was followed for 29 years. Because of their celibacy and abstinence from smoking, their mortality from prostatic cancer was found to be 29% and from lung cancer 41% lower. However, the mortality from cancer of the larynx and cirrhosis of the liver was 47% and diabetes 82% higher [22].

There are studies, however, that present opposite evidence. In the Caerphilly study, 918 men aged 45–59 years provided responses on the recalled number of orgasms. Within 10 years of follow up, 67 respondents died from coronary heart disease and 83 from other causes. Researchers concluded that,"Mortality risk in the group with high frequency of orgasm was less than half of that of the group with low frequency" [23]. A serious limitation of this study, however, is that it was based on the "recalled number of orgasms" which could be over exaggerated in the high frequency group.

In a study in Gothenburg, Sweden, 166 men and 226 women aged 70 were examined. Five years later 32 men and 23 women had died. The study found that, "There was a positive association in married men between mortality and early cessation of sexual intercourse" [24]. My explanation would be that men who ceased to perform their marital duties experienced a humiliation and neglect from their wives, became miserable and died of depression. When I see a nasty woman treating her husband as garbage, I suspect that he doesn't sexually satisfy her.

In my view, we are better off with lowering our testosterone level instead of increasing it, as you hear all around. Men around the world are obsessed with sex and pay for it dying prematurely. Conventional sex kills men, but those who have mastered an ejaculation control technique, live a long life as did Dr. Stanley Bass, author of the book, *Better than Orgasm* [25].

4. *Lose weight.* Go ketogenic. Restrict your carbohydrate intake [26]. Insulin, a hormone produced in our body in response to sugar and starchy food (and protein to some extent) is responsible for accelerated aging and a host of many diseases, such as diabetes, metabolic syndrome [27], heart disease, and stroke, just to name a few.

5. *Move south.* The closer to the equator you live, the longer your life is. Hilton Hotema's book is titled *Long Life In Florida* [28], not in Alaska. The highest ratio or prevalence of centenarians in Japan is found in Okinawa, a southern island, and not in north-eastern prefectures of Japan [29]. The detriments of living in the northern climates are discussed in more detail in Chapter 3.

6. *Move your body fat from your belly* back to under the skin, where it belonged when you were young. If you are not fond of liposuction therapies, a non-surgical alternative to liposuction is diet and exercise [30]. If your fat is under the skin, then increase your body fat content to 25% to match a woman's.

The health experts' attention is focused mostly on a weight loss but 1.5 million of American men are underweight [31]. Both being overweight and underweight undermines one's health and shortens their lifespan [32]. In the developed countries, elderly folks are more vulnerable of becoming underweight and malnourished (due to diseases) than other groups of population. In the study of 3,286 men and women aged 65 to 87 years in Tromsø, Norway, the health-related quality of life (HRQoL) was found to be lower in underweight subjects. "HRQoL was significantly reduced in elderly people at increased risk of malnutrition, and this was more pronounced in men than in women" [33]. A similar result regarding HRQoL scores was obtained in a study of male veterans by Arterburn DE, et al., who reported that ,"Scores of overweight patients (body mass index: 25 to 29.9 kg/m2) were higher (better) than those of normal weight patients in 11 domains" [34].

Skinny people can suffer decreased muscle and bone mass, impaired immune function, poor wound healing and pressure ulcers, just to name a few [35]. Being underweight, overweight, or obese is classified by the body mass index (BMI). To calculate BMI, a person's weight in pounds (lb) is divided by the height in inches squared $(in)^2$, and the result is multiplied by a factor of 703. In my case, BMI = 165 lb/$(74\ in)^2$ * 703 = 21,2.

In a study by Flegal KM, et al., mortality of underweight (BMI < 18) people over the age of 70 was found 69% greater than that for normal weight (BMI 18 to < 25) and 17% higher in obese (BMI ≥35) people [36]. Noteworthy that mortality in overweight (BMI 25 to < 30) cohort in this study was 9% lower than in normal weight group. The result for mortality of overweight people was consistent with the Cardiovascular Health Study, a population-based cohort study of 5888 older adults. Researchers concluded that, "…older adults who are overweight (or, in some cases, obese) have no worse and sometimes better outcomes than those of normal weight at 65" [37].

There are a few strategies of gaining weight well known in the bodybuilding and sumo wrestling world but the basic idea is to increase caloric intake by eating more food. Under-nourished individuals must gradually introduce more nutrition-dense foods including animal proteins and fats, starchy vegetables, and full-fat dairy products (for Blood type Bs). In a review article, *Underweight, the Less Discussed Type of Unhealthy Weight and Its Implications,* to gain weight, Stella G. Uzogara recommended: "The menu should include items such as lean meat, oily fish, poultry and eggs, legumes (beans and peas), milk, avocado, various nuts and seeds" [38]. In her expert advice, all items sound good to me accept for the "lean meat" which I believe will defeat the purpose. The fattier the meat, the better and it is more savory.

How much should one aim in weight gaining? As studies show, moderately overweight elderly people fare better that normal weight. Our target must be 25% body fat as normal weight women display. To calculate your current body fat, the body fat calculator will be helpful [39]. The input data contain weight, height, neck, waist, and hip circumference. By using this calculator, you can see the progress for your increasing weight and other parameters until you reach your target. For those of us who doubt if this amount of body fat is not excessive, the Mayo Clinic classifies for men 61-79 years old the 13-25% body fat as healthy [39].

The more desirable than just waist line fat is subcutaneous (under the skin) fat. It can be increased by having a nap after a weight-lifting exercise and meal, by taking cold shower and some other strategies [40].

7. *Avoid injuries and psychological trauma.* A severe head injury with fainting increases risk of Parkinson's disease (PD) as the 2013 meta-analysis of the 22 studies demonstrated [41]. This result was confirmed by the study of 235 PD cases and 464 controls in the island of Cyprus in the eastern Mediterranean in which the risk of PD was 94% higher than in controls. Noteworthy that lifestyle and environmental factors such as exposure to pesticides and eating more nuts, red meat and drinking more soft drinks increased the risk, whereas eating more fish and drinking wine decreased the PD risk [42].

Both physical and psychological trauma such as an accident or extremely stressful experience such as an abuse or loss of a spouse leaves us with an anxiety, depression of the spirit, insomnia, edginess, as well as an upset stomach. It can take a long time to recover and return to our normal condition. After some serious injuries, an abnormal function persists life-long. Forty years ago, when I was in my late thirties, I broke both bones of my left leg just above the ankle. I stepped on an ice ball covered with fresh snow, my foot twisted, and I fell. I didn't feel much pain and trying to get up, to my surprise, I couldn't because my leg was broken. An emergency vehicle brought me to the hospital where they drilled a hole through my heel bone, inserted a rod, and adjusted weights to it, which pulled my foot to align with my leg. I spent three weeks in the hospital lying on my back in an immobile position and was then discharged with a cast covering my leg up to above the knee.

Two crunches assisting me in moving around became my companions for about three months. After the cast, which had many funny jokes written with a marker by my friends, was taken off, I had hard time to make my knee bending again. Being immobile for a few months, uric acid deposits petrified my knee and I felt sharp pains with each attempt to bend it. I was persistent, though, and after another three months was able to jog and take a lotus or padmasana yoga posture, which is quite challenging for many people having even no leg injuries. But my left knee and ankle have never attained the ease with which I can bend the joints of my unaffected right leg due to damage to the cartilage.

My problem, however, is minor comparing with what happened to Eugeny, my school mate. He was born with a birth defect, his left leg was underdeveloped, non-functional, and just dangling from his hip. From the beginning of his life, he moved around with a support of a crunch and cane. At the time when we graduated from the high school, he looked very athletic in his upper torso, with a broad shoulders and muscular arms. In his early 20s, when he was a student of a medical school, getting out of the bus, he stumbled, fell and broke his only leg. Both bones in the middle section between a knee and ankle of his right leg (tibia and fibula bones) were broken. His treatment was not successful and he developed a false joint in the broken area. I imagine how much suffering he endured in his life.

In my case, I had more luck than Eugeny and many others. While in the hospital, my traumatologist doctor shared that in his practice, in two out of ten cases of broken limbs, by entirely unknown reasons, bones failed to heal, gangrene was developing, and limbs had to be amputated. Heavy cigarette smokers, even young men, can develop a condition called thromboangiitisobliterans (Buerger' disease), an inflammatory disease of the peripheral arteries. Inflammation is accompanied by the thrombus formation, and in advanced stage, can lead to gangrene [9, p.997-8]. The most important part in treatment is quitting smoking, but in many cases, people are so addicted to smoking that they fail it and face multiple amputations .

Another common condition that leads to amputations is diabetes. It is quite often these days to see people in a wheel chair with amputated legs. When I was selling my book as a street vendor in New York City about ten years ago, one artist selling his icon-like paintings had both his legs cut off. If you happened to take a bus in the New York City, at the stops the bus kneels to let people in wheel chairs without legs in and out. Noteworthy that Jan Kwasniewski, M.D. of Poland claims that his low carb, moderate protein, and high fat Optimal diet cures both the Buerger's disease and diabetes [43].

Thus, more than looking for entertainment or pleasures, we need to avoid harm of any kind. We are better off of driving safely and doing our daily activities in our home and out there with security and precautions. By all means, we need to avoid dangerous activities, physical exertions or a stressful situation.

8. *Avoid iatrogenic disease*, a disease caused by doctors, their prescriptions and procedures. Stay away from doctors, both allopathic and alternative, unless in case of emergency. Doctors are not bad guys, they just don't know the cause of person's illness and don't understand the unique type of their patients. Their drugs, antibiotics, and treatments all have strong side effects including death. Though regular medical checkups and non-invasive tests are necessary. though. Instead of relying on doctors, we need to take a good care of ourselves, invest our time and efforts in our health and fitness, and to become self-sufficient. Our goal is being free from help outside, unless it is absolutely necessary. This way we can reclaim ownership for our life. This is a sure way to be healthy and happy, and enjoy our life.

Take the advice of George H. Steele, MD, *"The Best Way to Stay Healthy: Stay as Far Away from Doctors as You Can"* [44]. Do your own research, become your own doctor as I do. In his bestselling book published in 2015, *How Not to Die*, Michael Greger, MD, has a special chapter, *How Not to Die from Iatrogenic Causes (or, How Not to Die from Doctors)*. He shares, "For example, side effects from medications given in hospitals kill an estimated 106,000 Americans every year. That statistic alone effectively makes medical care the sixth-leading cause of death in the United States" [45].

One can argue that this number based on the 1998 study by Lazarou, et al. [46] is outdated and way underestimated. At Johns Hopkins in 2016, "...the patient safety experts have calculated that more than 250,000 deaths per year are due to medical error in the U.S ...making it the third leading cause of death after heart disease and cancer" [47].

It has been reported in 2004 "that the total number of deaths caused by conventional medicine is an astounding 783,936 per year" [48, 49]. Dr. Christopher Kent commented that, "It is evident that the American medical system is the leading cause of death and injury in the United States" [50].

Greger, a medical doctor himself, has a solution for men (and for women), "The best way to avoid the adverse effects of medical tests and treatments is not to avoid doctors but to avoid getting sick in the first place" [45].

I agree, because in the case of emergency we need to see a doctor. As Greger puts it, "Doctors excel at treating acute conditions, such as mending broken bones and curing infections, but for chronic diseases, which are the leading causes of death and disability, conventional medicine doesn't have much to offer and, in fact, can sometimes do more harm than good" [45].

Men usually smoke more and for longer periods in their lives than women and develop conditions such as cardiovascular disease or lung problems caused by excessive smoking. Nowadays everyone knows that cigarette smoking is detrimental to our health, causing cardiovascular diseases (CVD) and many cancers. "Tobacco smoke oxidizes cholesterol by both introducing and increasing the generation of free radicals within your body. Both damaged cholesterol and increased free-radical production increase the rate of arterial plaque formation" [51, p.101], thus leading to CVD.

If you smoke cigarettes, which are loaded with carcinogens, your immune system is compromised. Mikkel Schmidt, however, in his reply to comments of Davey Jones on the immune system followed the speech of Global health expert Alanna Shaikh on the TED show on March 11, 2020, about the Covid-19 coronavirus outbreak suggests that "the most effective way to avoid getting infected, if we look at the data from China and the US, is to start smoking (smokers are extremely underrepresented in Covid-19 cases), but it will be way worse for you in the long run" [52]. However, these claims were not confirmed in the meta-analysis conducted on May 12, 2020, which stated that, "...the available evidence suggests that smoking is associated with increased severity of disease and death in hospitalized Covid-19 patients" [53].

I would agree if non-smokers start smoking not cigarettes but real tobacco cigars or pipe tobacco. The smoke of a cigar is too strong to inhale and you will just puff. In doing so, you will sanitize your mouth and will swallow with the saliva nicotine known also as a nicotinic acid, niacin, or Vitamin B3, which is very healthy. George Burns never smoked cigarettes but smoked 5-6 cigars a day and lived to the age of 100. Starting smoking at the age of 14, by some estimates, he smoked around 140,000 cigars in his lifetime [54].

When admitted to the hospitals, men die more often "than women who suffer from the same chronic conditions, implying that men may experience more-severe forms of these conditions" [55]. A healthy lifestyle plus good eating habits outlined in my books is a way not to become sick.

9. Go hairless, not wireless. Men can learn this secret from women who do not grow hair on their face. Before puberty (becoming sexually mature), boys and girls have no body hair. Under the influence of sex hormones, e.g. estrogen in females and testosterone in males, they grow hair in their pubic area and their facial and body hair in men. Some men grow a lot of hair on their chest, and their arms, legs, and even the back can become quite hairy.

Growing hair involves a synthesis of keratin protein, which requires growth factors in addition to sex hormones, such as growth hormone, which is physiological before puberty and becomes pathological thereafter. After puberty is achieved, the aging process kicks in and growth hormone is an aide to it.

Men who take synthetic growth hormone to increase muscle mass put themselves into precarious position of growing a tumor. Bigger muscles are impressive but nothing good in life comes without the price tag attached to it. The tradeoff of becoming muscular can be a decreased longevity.

The greatest role model for men is naked mole rats. Aside from not growing hair, what other secrets can naked mole rats share with men? Breathing in less oxygen and accumulating more carbon dioxide in their system is probably the most powerful means for life extension [56]. To protect themselves against predators such as snakes, they plug the entrances into their burrows and breathe less oxygenated air.

In our aerobic environment, we depend on oxygen for all metabolic processes, but oxygen is an aging agent 007 imposing oxidative stress and gradually but steadily damages all our tissues and organs. The long living people in some "longevity valleys," such as Abkhazia in Georgia, Hunza in Pakistan and Vilcabamba in Ecuador (despite their age exaggeration) dwelling in the mountains, breathe in thin air low in oxygen and burn themselves out slower than at the sea level.

10. Learn from the zebrafish. Another role model for men after naked mole rats is zebrafish (*Daniorerio*), a tiny (2 to 3 inch long) and robust freshwater fish which is distributed in India, Pakistan, Bangladesh, Nepal, Myanmar, and Bhutan. Zebrafish inhibit in slow moving or stagnant waters such as streams, rivers, ponds, ditches, and rice fields. Zebrafish is a popular aquarium fish, known as Zebra Danio.

In their genetic structure, zebrafish resembles by 70 per cent our genes and by 84 per cent the genes associated with human disease. Major body systems, organs and tissues such as blood, muscle, kidney and eyes in zebrafish are similar to those in humans. Humans have an ability to regenerate skeletal muscle and large parts of the liver [57] but zebrafish is superior to us as they know how to repair the injured heart muscle and as fast as within a few weeks [58]. Aside of the heart, an adult zebrafish can regrow injured or amputated tissues which include retinae and optic nerves of the eye, brain, spinal cord, fins, pancreas, liver, and kidney [59].

Zebrafish does this by utilizing progenitor or stem cells derived from their own tissues [60]. Regenerative ability by means of stem cells is not limited to zebrafish alone. Other animals are also capable of tissue regeneration, e. g., the Xenopus tadpole can regenerate the tail [61], amphibians can grow new limbs [62], and urodele (newt, salamander and axolotl) and anuran (frogs and toads) amphibians can grow new neurons and glia cells thus regenerating the brain [63]. Urodele amphibians can also regenerate spinal cord, limb, retina, and lens of the eyes [60]. Although histological (microscopic structure on a cellular level) composition of the heart of zebrafish is similar to that of other vertebrates, its adult heart, with one atrium and one ventricle, is simpler and smaller (about 1 mm^3) than the mammalian heart. Furthermore, as recent research shows, "Myocardial regeneration in zebrafish is not based on stem cells or transdifferentiation of other cell types but on the proliferation of preexisting cardiomyocytes" [64].

Many people die having a heart attack called myocardial infarction (MI) caused by the thrombus (blood clot) formation and blockage of a coronary artery. In those lucky ones who survive a heart attack, as a consequence of prolonged myocardial ischemia (reduced blood flow to the heart), the left ventricle muscle is damaged (cardiomyocyte death primarily by necrosis) and irreversibly lost. Functional contractile myocardium is replaced with a non-contractile scar resulting in a diminished heart ejection function. In these people, there is a likelihood of progression to congestive heart failure and premature death. The story is different with zebrafish which, after surgical resection of about 20% of the cardiac ventricle, establish a transient fibrotic scar that within 2 months is progressively replaced with new myocardial tissue and newly formed blood vessels. This regrown cardiac muscle is contractile and fully functional [65].

Is it something specific in the zebrafish diet which can explain its unsurpassed regeneration power? It is primarily omnivorous fish feeding on brine shrimp, bloodworms and zooplankton like mosquito and its larvae, live insects such as daphnia (planktonic crustaceans), cyclops (water flea), tubifex worms, and invertebrate eggs. The zebrafish diet, though, includes also phytoplankton, algae, plant material, and spores. [66]. Other small fish in the same rivers and ponds probably feed on a similar fare but doesn't possess extra abilities as zebrafish have. In his advertisement video, Andy Perth exploits the fame of zebrafish by selling supplements such as VisiClear for eyesight improvement and claiming that he restored his vision from being nearly blind to 20/20. His formula allegedly stimulates the production of the adult repair stem cells which zebrafish utilizes for regeneration of various organs and tissues. The ingredients, based on the zebrafish diet, include Lutein, Zeoxanthin, Astaxanthin, L-carnitine, Bladderack, Grapeseed extract, Blueberry extract, Resviratrol, and Spirulina [67]. However, Perth mistakenly asserts that zebrafish is a marine fish that inhibits the waters of Southeast Asia, hence Spirulina (marine algae) and Bladderack (seaweed) are in his formula. Indeed, all ingredients including carotenoids, Lutein, Zeoxanthin, and Astaxanthin, which decrease the risk of age-related macular degeneration and antioxidants Grapeseed extract, Blueberry extract, and Resviratrol are good for our eyes and health in general and probably will work to our benefit. But is it really its diet which makes zebrafish a role model of macular regeneration? Or is it its living environment?

An important feature noteworthy of mentioning is that zebrafish live in a low oxygen aquatic environment, their heart is highly adopted to hypoxia, and is capable of regeneration. The human or mouse, chicken, sheep embryo also develops in low-oxygen environment, but after birth the newborn's heart is exposed to the high-oxygen concentrations, and humans or other mammals loose the regeneration power. "Consequently it appears that species with cardiac regenerative capacity reside in a hypoxic environment" [68]. Among 64,000 vertebrates living on Earth that have the heart, only a dozen of species having heart regeneration ability were studied. Adult zebrafish, Giant Danio, Goldfish, and some amphibians can repair the heart after injury. The embryos of mammals including humans also can, but in an adult stage they lose this ability. As mentioned above, the clue might be the amount of oxygen that their heart is adapted to [69].

If naked mole rats, zebrafish and long-living people in the "longevity valleys" have common feature, its name is hypoxia. Naked mole rats who live in the underground burrows in the eastern Africa breathe in an air with 6% of O_2 [70]. Zebrafish in its natural habitat obtains oxygen dissolved in water via its gills. Under normal atmospheric pressure called normoxic, it is estimated that, in the ambient water, oxygen content is 7.5 mg of O_2 /L or 80 mm Hg [71], which translates to 10.4% of O_2. The "longevity valleys" dwellers of Vilcabamba, Ecuador and of Abkhazia, Georgia, live at altitude of 5,000 ft. (1,524 m) and of Hunza, Pakistan, at 8,000 ft (2,438 m). The effective oxygen of the air at the described altitudes is 17.3% and 15.4% respectively, as compared to 20.9% at sea level [72]. In the USA, two cities in the state of Colorado have similar elevations: Boulder 5,430 ft (1,655 m) and Aspen 7,908 ft (2,410 m). By their altitude, these two cities equate the longevity areas, but their latitude is a bit to the North. Vilcabamba (-4.3° S), Abkhazia (34.2° N), and Hunza (36.3° N) are closer to the Equator than Boulder, CO (40.0° N) and Aspen, CO (39.2° N).

From these comparisons we can conclude that probably high oxygen is the problem. Oxygen is a doubled-edge sword, it gives life to us, poor aerobic creatures, by one hand and takes it away slowly and steadily by another. With all our superiority over other animal co-inhabitants, we even don't know how to repair our heart without drastic bypass surgery or to repair our knees without replacing them with titanium ones.

The way out is to muse over oxygen issue more seriously. The less oxygen we breathe in, the healthier our heart is and the longer we live. In a 15-year-long study of 504 men and 646 women living in one mountainous and two lowland villages in Greece, those who lived at high altitudes (950 m) had less heart disease and all cause mortality than their lowland counterparts. "Residence in mountainous areas seems to have a "protective effect" from total and coronary mortality. Increased physical activity from walking on rugged terrains under conditions of moderate hypoxia among the mountain residents could explain these findings" [73].

In the United States, the highest altitude is in the state of Colorado, which is "considered to be one of the healthiest states, with low rates of obesity, cancer and heart disease" [74]. What is the better place for a man to live in: high altitude (mountains) or low latitude (south)? Both, I guess. Some Americans enjoy both worlds living in tropical countries like Costa Rico, Ecuador, and Colombia.

11. Move your body, exercise your brain. Do resistance, aerobic, breathing and flexibility exercises such as yoga. Long lived people are slim and trim. Walking or hiking are good examples of aerobic exercise. While living in the state of Maine, I used to hike on the nearby hill, even in the winter time on the snow wearing non-slippery boots. In Florida, where I live now, I walk for a half an hour every morning. To add to the intensity of my walking, I carry a backpack with a heavy dictionary in it. While walking, I inhale on four steps, exhale on four steps, and stop breathing on the next eight steps. If the car passes by, I stop breathing for 20 or so seconds and then grasp a fresh air. A few more people in our 55+ community are walking enthusiasts but they don't use my breath-holding trick and inhaling the exhaust fumes do more harm to their body than good.

Resistant training is very popular and many people go to gym and spend an hour or more with their workouts. Ordinarily, they "pump iron" with free weights or using machines doing many repetitions and sets to all-out fatigue state. Over years they definitely achieve some results with building muscles and reducing body fat. However, much more efficient and markedly less time consuming is a negative training method developed by Ellington Darden, Ph.D. [75]. With this resistant training technique, the lifting part of the repetition (positive training) is secondary, and the lowering (negative) part is emphasized. I do the lowering phase of a pushup for 24 sec (goal 30 sec) three times or lowering 20 lb. dumbbells in each hand for 30 sec two times and that's it. Stepping on the rubber resistance band, side-raising hands and then lowering them for 30 sec is an exercise for shoulders that I do too. After each exercise, my muscles involved feel sore indicating that some training effect is achieved.

You can exercise your brain by memorizing holy books, prayers, reciting poems, learning a foreign language, anatomy, physiology, mathematics or playing piano, organ and other musical instruments.

12. Cleanse and purify yourself. Avoid pollutants and rid of toxins and parasites. Multiple pollutions: air, water, food, EMF, sound pollution and acidifying food all put a great stress on our elimination organs. We suffer of constipation, toxic liver, gallbladder, liver, kidneys and bladder stones, slugged lymphatic system and clogged arteries. Go to the sauna, you need to sweat to expel toxins from your body. Enemas for colon cleanse, liver-gallbladder flush, kidneys flush, lymph and blood vessels cleanse can be done at your home.

Sick and toxic people around us make us sick. Not only that we can be infected with the air born viruses or bacteria or sexually transmitted diseases but irritable and angry people create a toxic environment around them. "Whether it's negativity, cruelty, the victim syndrome, or just plain craziness, toxic people drive your brain into a stressed-out state that should be avoided at all costs" [76]. Medical and health care professionals are even in a worse situation than most of us since it is their job to deal with sick people on a daily basis. If they will find time in their busy schedule to read this book, they will definitely benefit from it.

13. Become a self-healer to heal yourself from inside out. Most people have a mindset that in case of illness they need to find someone else, e.g. medical or alternative doctor, nutrition adviser, yoga teacher, spiritual guru, etc. They look for help from others. Very few know that each of us has a tremendous inner power to produce all necessary biochemical substances within ourselves. We have the potential to unearth a dormant pharmaceutical factory and generate all hormones, enzymes, and bioactive molecules capable of curing our ailments.

One of those who knew how to do it was Russian scientist, Georgy N. Sytin, MD, (1921-2016). He called his approach, "a method of the volitional control of a person's state by the use of emotionally charged words and mental images" [77]. It is based on the teachings of Ivan P. Pavlov (1849-1936), a prominent Russian physiologist and psychologist, who viewed speech as a second signal system (words are signal of signals) in its relation to the subconsciousness governing physiological processes of the body [78]. Pavlov was a Nobel Prize winner in Physiology or Medicine in 1904.

According to Sytin, "...our thoughts are material, consisting of a spiritual matter, which in its organization is higher and stronger than physical matter and has an unlimited effect on physical matter, including the matter of the physical body of a person" [79]. Although invisible, "Thoughts, emotions, desires, our mental states, they all generate a field around us" [80], like electric, gravitation, or magnetic fields.

Thoughts are powerful energy and it is proved by the ability of some psychics "...to move physical objects by sheer mind power" [81], a phenomenon which is known as telekinesis. The Oxford Dictionary defines telekinesis as "The supposed ability to move objects at a distance by mental power or other nonphysical means" [82].

Edgar D. Mitchell (1930-2016), an American NASA astronaut who, after returning from the moon, became interested in parapsychology and founded the Institute of Noetic Sciences. Describing the telekinesis experiments in that institute with Uri Geller, an Israeli psychic, Mitchell said, "We've watched him change the readings on an electronic pan-balance . . . both increasing the weight and levitating a one-gram mass – getting very nice spikes on it, indicating that there is an impulse in both the downward direction and then, at a later time, in the upward direction. A very significant experiment" [81]. Dr. Mitchell, who held a Sc. D. (post-doctoral) degree in aeronautics from the Massachusetts Institute of Technology (MIT), considered this experiment as proof of Geller's telekinetic ability.

Currently, in physics and related sciences, telekinesis (psychokinesis) is not considered a real phenomenon and is generally regarded as pseudoscience [82]. However, Mitchell's experiment with positive results is not mentioned in the Wikipedia articles on psychokinesis [83] or Uri Geller [84] which leaves me with an impression of these two articles being biased focusing only on experiments with negative outcomes.

Letting neuroscientists argue whether our mind is generating thoughts or receiving them from outer sources [80], we will agree with Swami Vivekananda who stated that, "Thought is a force, as is gravitation or repulsion"[86]. Words represent or reflect our thoughts. Words encode a mental picture (or a thought) that others can understand. In conversation, we use words to communicate our thoughts to others.

Georgy N. Sytin developed a method of "...healing-rejuvenation by creative thoughts (healing moods), assimilating which, each person can defeat any ailments, resist age-related changes and significantly extend his life" [87]. Sytin's method of verbal, image-shaped, emotionally-charged volitional self-conviction includes thought, words, emotion, and will. His verbal formulas (moods) act like mantras. "Will is a kind of thought that carries a command with authority" [88]. Sytin's moods are directed at an individual who creates a mental image of themselves as a young, healthy, strong, beautiful, and ever-improving person. Their ills and ailments are looked at as temporary conditions which will be quickly overcome. The session involves "... self-persuasion through reading or listening to positive affirmations (self-tuning verbal formulas)" [89]. The mood is a precisely formulated thought of a person about themselves, to influence the physical body and psyche, aimed to improve health, heal, and rejuvenate. Sytin's moods are "...unique texts with a specially selected set of phrases aimed at activating the brain, which then gives a powerful impulse to the body, to the organs, practically ordering the diseased organ to heal, to return to its original healthy state" [90]. To overcome a serious health condition, the session could be as long as four hours a day but one to two hours is necessary for prevention.

The power of words for self-healing has been earlier recognized by Emile Coué (1857-1926), a French pharmacist and psychologist, who developed a method of the "mantra-like conscious suggestion," known as autosuggestion, at the beginning of the 20 th century [91]. Coué's verbal formula, "Every day, in every way, I'm getting better and better," is well recognized. Coué advised to routinely repeat this formula 20 times daily, early in the morning and in the evening of each day. Concerning to self-healing a particular condition, "...if a person firmly believes that his or her asthma is disappearing, then this may happen, as far as the body is able physically to overcome or control the illness" [92]. He strongly advised us to focus on and imagine desired, positive results and avoid negative thoughts about one's health, because mind and body may accept this thought and an illness could develop.

Likewise, Sytin realized that creating an image for a person that they are healthy, young, and strong and see themselves this way at present and decades ahead in the future, will bring about the best results in self-healing and rejuvenation. Sytin maintained that in this case, the nervous system will organize the work of the mind and body in such a way that person will remain healthy, young, and strong in the future. In a support of this idea, Sytin relied on theories of "feedback" and "functional systems," elaborated by Pyotr K. Anokhin (1898-1974), a distinguished Russian biologist and physiologist who created his theories under the guidance of Ivan Pavlov [93]. Anokhin was regarded as a scientist who built a bridge between physiology and psychology.

Both Coué and Sytin had great success in curing patients with various physical and mental conditions. Coué, being a pharmacist, never claimed to be a healer; however a list of ailments, that he helped people with, "...included kidney problems, diabetes, memory loss, stammering, weakness, atrophy, and all sorts of physical and mental illnesses [92]. Sytin, who was a medical doctor, mentioned in one of his Russian TV interviews the successful healing of his patients with multiple sclerosis, infantile paralysis, schizophrenia, impotence, fibroids of the uterus, different types of mastopathy, cysts on the ovaries, prostate adenoma (enlargement), and migraine, just to name a few.

Examples of Sytin moods are:

"I live a divinely beautiful, joyful, happy life. With the brightness of lightning, I see myself in the future, in 100 years, and in 300 years and beyond, in the prime of my divinely beautiful youth. I clearly see myself at the beginning of my life. My whole life is ahead of me."

"With every passing minute, nerves are getting healthier and stronger throughout my body. I am born a man of nerves of steel. Newborn life gives birth to me as a newborn-young hero of a powerful physique."

"In thirty years, and in fifty years, and in a hundred years I will remain cheerful and indestructibly healthy young person full of health and strength" [94].

Unlike psychic healer Anatoly Kashpirovsky, 81, a Russian psychotherapist of Ukrainian origin [95], who claimed to be able to tap into the inner resources and reverse health conditions that were once thought irreversible, both Coué and Sytin urged one to tap into their inner resources with their "help-yourself" method, using one's willful self-convicting suggestions or affirmations (moods).

Everyone knows that words can hurt. One of my friends would become sick and depressed for days after being exposed to someone's scathing remark. As Pavlov implied, "Words can be a stimulus (irritant) for a man similar to physical irritants for animals." On the flip side, words have the power to heal.

Verbal suggestions were found to be helpful with a few somatic (pertaining to sensations) symptoms such as pain, itch, dyspnea (breathlessness), fatigue, and nausea, as the 2019 study review show [96]. In a study of ten women with mild sleep complaints. "...an inert compound, administered with the suggestion that it was a hypnotic substance" markedly improved the quality of their sleep [97]. In another study of 60 healthy subjects, the verbal suggestion of analgesia (absence of a normal sense of pain) led to "...a significant increase in pain tolerance." In the same study, ten Parkinson's patients demonstrated a better motor performance after a verbal suggestion was administered [98]. One more condition that verbal suggestion is effective for is depression [99].

Noteworthy that Satin strongly advocated avoiding such words as ache or pain, especially with headaches. He shared that some people trying to "improve" his moods, as they thought, would repeatedly utter, "I have no headache, I have no headache." However, instead of diminishing, a headache would greatly increase to the extent that they would end up with migraines. His idea had been proved valid a few years later by a study of 16 healthy subjects (8 males and 8 females) at Jena University in Germany. The functional magnetic resonance tomography (fMRT) was used for brain imaging. The study psychologists observed a neuronal activation in pain-related brain areas in response to pain words. "Our results indicate that pain-related words activate regions associated with the pain matrix, especially when subjects were explicitly attending to words," researchers concluded [100].

To eliminate headache, Sytin advised creating a mental picture of a head being vast, weightless, and bright, filled with light, and having a vigorous blood circulation. "All arteries of the head are Divinely expanded, Divinely free along their entire length. Through all the arteries, arterioles, capillaries, and veins of the head, blood flows in a free, wide, joyful stream. Through all the arterioles of the head, overall the capillaries of the head, blood flows in a wide, free spring stream, like a cheerful spring river in a flood, in a wide flood." This mental image improves blood circulation and usually, according to Sytin, headache disappears in a matter of minutes.

Dr. Sytin was living proof of the effectiveness of his method. In the combat during World War II, at the age of 23, he was nine times wounded; the last combat injury was considered mortal by his doctors—a shrapnel had entered his abdomen and lodged in his backbone destroying his spinal nerves. Doctors even didn't want to operate on him deeming him helpless. However, he made it through the night repeating non-stop, "The volitional effort. The volitional effort. The bleeding stops. The bleeding stops. I will survive. I will survive. I am getting better. I am getting better." The next day he was found still alive, doctors operated on him and he completely recovered a few years later. Sytin was inhumanly productive: he won four D.Sc. (post-gradual) degrees in medicine, psychology, philosophy, and pedagogy, wrote 200 books and received patients until he died at the age of 95. He had four children and his last son, Oleg, was born when Sytin was 70 years old.

Affirmations are even helpful in releasing "feel-good" substances, such as serotonin, dopamine, and endorphins. "Research shows that up to 80 percent of the thoughts we produce in a day is negative, and you can't live a positive life with a negative mind. Affirmations are proven methods of self-improvement because of their ability to re-wire our brains by increasing the level of endorphins released into the body" [101]. In scary times like the current coronavirus pandemic, positive affirmations can help to avoid fear and anxiety. "Writing down positive affirmations right when you wake up or before going to bed can also be very powerful in rewiring your mindset," tells Dr. Janine Kreft [102], an Austin-based clinical psychologist [103].

14. Don't be afraid of the corona virus and thus allowing a corona virus egregore to drain your energy. What is an egregore? The Theosophy Wiki defines egregore as "a group thought-form. It can be created intentionally or unintentionally and becomes an autonomous entity with the power of influence" [104]. As an occult concept, an egregore is a "collective group mind, an autonomous psychic entity made up of and influencing the thoughts of the group of people" [105]. The like-minded group like a family, a club, a corporation, a political party, a religion, prayer group, church, or cult, a fad in popular culture, or a state and country can create egregore with their collective thought, volitional effort, and visualization. "An egregore is a kind of group mind which is created when people consciously come together for a common purpose" [106].

The concept of an egregore ("watcher" in the Ancient Greek language) was familiar to people in ancient Greece and Rome who imagined them as "observant angels" watching over their cities. In the contemporary usage, in the Russian spiritual book, "Roza Mira" (Rose of the World), by Daniil Andreev, the notion of egregore "...represents the shining cloud-like spirit associated with the Church" [105]. Like any other energy, e. g., light, sound, electricity, or magnetism, every human thought exists in the form of energy waves with a specific wavelength and frequency. "Quantum physics teaches us there is no difference between energy and matter" [107]. Identical thoughts of like-minded people (religious, political, sports, etc.), vibrate on the same wavelength and with the same frequency. By the law of resonance, these thoughts are amplified, a transfer of the subtle energy takes place, and they flow from an emitting source (people) into a psychic, subtle-energy field (receiver). Thus an energy-information field on the mental plane is created which is called egregore.

Is the egregore a real phenomenon? Most likely you are a person who is unacquainted with it and never heard about it. I don't expect you to be an esoteric believer and the term "egregore" may sound not palatable to you. Some recent Internet occult contributors colored it with dark colors. I do not consider myself to be New Age adept, though, but I do not see anything fearful in egregores. However, if this is the case for you, please take it as a metaphor. Furthermore, to accept the concept of the egregore, one has to overcome the intrinsic human materialistic skepticism.

"Egregores are energy-informational bodies, involuntarily created by human thought, omnipresent structures of colossal complexity and power, invisibly controlling all actions of humanity and feeding on them" [106].

For its existence, an egregore relies upon the devotion of a group of people, which sustains it by their believes and rituals that are usually emotionally charged. For instance, some members of a big family belong to a church, other ones are the members of a political party, and yet other members belong to a golf or tennis club. A few adult members work for one or more corporations. These egregores are a part of a larger country egregore which is the egregore of Italy where this family lives. Although the intentions with which these egregores have been created were good, each of these egregores competes with other egregores to steal their members to take their energy.

Since egregores are created by a collective group mind and, after attaining enough power, become an autonomous psychic entity, their mystery lies in their invisibility. They are invisible as our thoughts are, for most people, though. However, some advanced yogi masters, like Eugene Bazh, my former yoga teacher, can see the body of thought with their third eye. Twice upon a time, when we were together, I prepared a tricky question for him. Before I uttered it, he recognized it by saying, "You will ask me now a bad question." He explained that he saw an ugly brownish-colored thought to flow into my head. For me, it was proof that the thought is material and can be seen.

The substance of egregores, which exist on the mental plane is energy and information supplied to them by the members of the group. The "mental plane" or "world of thought" in the New Age philosophy is "...a macrocosmic or universal plane or reality that is made up purely of thought or mind stuff" [108]. That is where egregores belong and they were around as long as humanity.

The variety, shape, and size of egregores are huge: egregores represent various professions, religions, nations, peoples' beliefs, skills, interests, habits, states, emotions, desires, obsessions, and so forth. An example of a professional egregore is the "healing egregore." Physicians, medicine men, and folk healers of all times and nations have been concerned with curing and preventing diseases in the best possible way: remedies, drugs, surgeries, herbs, healthy food, lifestyle, and so on. Their thoughts have formed the "healing egregore," which exists in the mental plane. In a physical plane, each country has a medical organization, and globally, there is the World Health Organization (WHO) established in 1948 which purpose is to help all people on earth to attain good health. However, the medical thought on earth has existed from the beginning of time and its counterpart on the mental plane is "healing egregore." Doctors and healers around the world are its members, although the overwhelming majority of them have no slightest idea about that. Nevertheless, each member of this invisible organization unwillingly exchanges energy and information with an egregore.

In medicine or any other profession, among the majority of professionals, few are true devotees, who allocate most of their time and mental effort to their trade. They get in a close connection with their egregore which receives good supplies of energy from them and, in return, allows them to access its "information storage room." The egregore grants these rare individuals with discoveries, inventions, and flow of new ideas [102]. Such a professional works very hard over, say, the scientific problem thus establishing a connection channel with egregore and then, usually in their trans-like state, dream, or daydream, receives an insight into discovery or invention. That is how Friedrich A. Kekulé (1829-1896), a German organic chemist [109], described his discovery of a benzene ring-shaped molecule, "...after having a reverie or day-dream of a snake seizing its own tail" [110].

Another example of tapping into an egregore of chemistry is Dmitri I. Mendeleev (1834-1907), a Russian chemist and discoverer of the periodic table. He "...claimed to have envisioned the complete arrangements of the elements in a dream." He wrote, "I saw in a dream a table where all elements fell into place as required. Upon awakening, I immediately wrote it down on a piece of paper" [111]. Yet another example is Nicola Tesla (1856-1943), a Serbian-American inventor, best known for his invention of the alternating current (AC), electric car, and his works on free energy. He often had visions which "...provided the solution to a particular problem he had encountered." Tesla would "...visualize an invention in his mind with extreme precision" [112]. Even famous Albert Einstein (1879-1955), a German-born theoretical physicist, a developer of the theory of General Relativity, allegedly postulated his theory having an insight in his childhood dream. In his dream, he saw a herd of electrocuted cows jumping in the air and his arguments with cows farmer who saw what happened to cows differently. Inspired to meditate upon the dream's meaning, he came up with a "...conception of space and time, arguing that the relationship between the two is relative" [113], hence his theory of relativity was born.

Should egregores be regarded as Gods (good), Demons (bad), or Dictators (ugly)? [114]. On the "good" side, egregore can be beneficial to each member of the group. Egregore "...continuously interacts with its members, influencing them and being influenced by them. The interaction works positively by stimulating and assisting its members but only as long as they behave and act in line with its original aim" [115]. Also, in his book, "*Egregores: The Occult Entities That Watch Over Human Destiny*," Mark Stavish shares: "An egregore that receives enough sustenance can take on a life of its own, becoming an independent deity with powers its believers can use to further their spiritual advancement and material desires" [116]. Egregores will support and protect their adherents, to provide them with energy and information, and to influence all aspects of their life in the desired way.

On the "bad" side, egregores can harm and hurt those who disobey or rebel. The independent thinking of a member of the group can be compromised, because of "...an ever-present danger of group-think taking over one's outlook on life." In his article on egregores. W. E. Butler has warned that the egregore's "...energy can be used for good or evil purposes" and "unless care is taken the power of independent thought may be reduced." [117]. I don't think that denial of their potential harm, like "...no evidence that soul-sucking cosmic leeches are trying to drain our energy" [118] will make us any good. For an ignorant person, they are dangerous, because they "...suppress the free actions of the personality, replacing them with the herd aspirations of the crowd" [108].

The coronavirus egregore most likely would fit into an "ugly" category. The mass hysteria created by the media sent waves of fear and anxiety around the globe that undeniably formed a psychic entity in the collective consciousness. Those who were afraid of coronavirus, focused on it and were talking about it contributed to the development of a coronavirus egregore. In her video, "How to modify the vibrations of the coronavirus egregore," Mindfulness Fani says, "Everyone is afraid of it, every single person, is responsible for creating it, this egregore of coronavirus. I know that it's hard to accept this but once you accepted it, you will know how to avoid it, and you will know how to stop it, not to create it, not give it power" [119]. Feeding off the people's fear and worries made it very powerful while depriving the whole nations of their vital energy.

What should we do? As one method, Mindfulness Fani suggested expressing gratitude to the Universe by saying, "Thank you!" a few times, especially upon awakening and before going to bed. Thank the Universe for the opportunity to modify vibrations of the egregore. To prevent your energy from being drained, Andres Leon of Columbia advises to detach oneself from a specific egregore, to ignore it. However, one needs to be aware of the concept of egregore and brave enough to go against it [120].

Fears and anxiety of people are fueled when they see that doctors don't know how to treat coronavirus disease: there are no effective medicines and no vaccines. Doctors, nurses, and other medical professionals are helpless themselves and they are dying by hundreds along with their patients [121]. By far, medical science and practice have offered three interventions: wash your hands with soap, wear a mask, and isolate yourself from others. Left alone and in despair, people search the Internet for alternative and home remedies. Earthclinic.com website shares success stories of people around the world. As one remedy, drinking an aspirin and lemon tea is suggested [122]. Other alternative treatments aiming to strengthen an immune system include Ayurveda, acupressure, coconut oil and essential oils, vitamins, minerals, detox, dietary changes with the emphasis of avoiding sugars, and simple carbohydrates which feed pathogens, etc. [123].

In the same line of home remedies fit "A method for the prevention and treatment of coronavirus disease at its early stage by destroying the virus in the nasopharynx by exposure to high temperatures," proposed

Prof. Yudin Gennady V., D Sc. in medicine from Ivanovo, Russia. He notes that "Covid-19 is an RNA molecule coated with a lipid (fatty) membrane. At a temperature of +60 °C (140 °F), it dies in 10 minutes." In this method, one brings to boil 1quart of water with 1 Tbsp of baking soda (to dissolve in alkaline medium its lipid membrane), bents over the pot, and inhales vapors of 80-90 °C (176-194 °F) for 15 min. Although other Russian doctors refute it [124], the combination of high temperature and alkaline environment sounds making sense to me. Velisar Rill, MD, a US cardiologist specializing in a Cardiac Catheterization [125], also refutes it, warning: "The problem is that the high temperature of the water vapors is intolerable to the nasopharynx; don't try it, it will burn the mucosa and tissues away." I will take his warning seriously and if I am to try it, I will stand high over the boiling water to avoid possible burning.

Of all factors increasing the vulnerability to Covid-19, the most prominent is the person's age. For elderly Covid-19 patients, a ketogenic (high fat) diet seems to improve clinical outcomes [126]. In its high-fat content, my "Blood Type A1 diet" [127] resembles the ketogenic diet. It emphasizes the use of healthy fats such as coconut oil, butter, ghee, and beef or lamb fat. Blood Type A1 is the most vulnerable to Covid-19 coronavirus of all blood types [128].

To fight effectively Covid-19 coronavirus, a healthy diet and lifestyle must include elements of Energy Medicine [105], which combines the physiology-targeted technologies of Western medicine with the psychology-oriented, subtle energy technologies of Oriental medicine, such as reflexology, Tai Chi, yoga, guided imagery, chakra energy, meditation, and affirmations. I believe that Sytin's affirmation which enhances an immune system, "With every passing moment, my immune system is strengthened millions of times. With gigantic Divine energy, it kills, destroys all viruses, all pathogenic microbes in all my internal organs and my entire body" [94], could be of great help.

3

LATITUDE AND HEART DISEASE CONNECTION

As it was mentioned earlier, living in warmer zones is beneficial to our health. Underexposure to the sun in the northern climates impairs the production of vitamin D in our skin. "In patients with multiple sclerosis, rheumatoid arthritis, and inflammatory bowel disease, deficiencies in vitamin D have been associated with an increased risk of disease activity"[129].

Vitamin D deficiency is traditionally not considered a risk factor for cardiovascular disease or all-cause mortality [130]. However there is a strong correlation between heart disease and low vitamin D levels and the traditional view is being challenged [131]. As stated in an article, *Vitamin D Deficiency and Risk for Cardiovascular Disease,* "Cross-sectional studies have reported that vitamin D deficiency is associated with increased risk of CVD, including hypertension, heart failure, and ischemic heart disease" [132]. In an investigation of "… 1739 Framingham Offspring Study participants (mean age 59 years; 55% women; all white) without prior cardiovascular disease," their "Vitamin D status was assessed by measuring 25-dihydroxyvitamin D (25-OH D)…" It was found that for levels <10 ng/m, CVD risk was 80% higher [133].

Dr. Rill is a firm advocate of the Vitamin D supplementation for cardiovascular health. He shares, "I can tell you that some of the lowest ever vitamin D levels (single digits) were in a patient with heart attacks and severe atherosclerotic burden. I was giving lectures 15 years ago showing slides of older women with low vitamin D levels, suffering from osteoporosis in spite of taking calcium supplements. The calcium was there but in the wrong place, in coronary arteries. Boron is also a very important and neglected cofactor in aberrance of calcium metabolism. Myself, I have been supplementing with vitamin D for 15 years at megadoses."

It is also suggested that, "UV radiation, by increasing body levels of vitamin D, protects against CVD by decreasing the risk of thrombus formation" [134]. The level of UV radiation increases in summer, in lower latitudes (closer to the equator), and elevated altitudes (high in the mountains). Many Western countries, Russia, northern China and Japan are located at higher latitudes, far north from the equator, where sun rays reach them at an angle, which decreases UV radiation and it effectiveness in synthesizing vitamin D in the skin.

It seems that the north or south can affect cardiovascular mortality in a particular country and across countries and continents. A study in Russia in 2009 found that the CVD mortality in the Northwest regions of Pskov (latitude 57.8° N) and Tver (56.8° N) were 1284 and 1263 deaths per 100,000 population, respectively. In the southern regions of Chechnya and Ingushetia (both 43.3° N), the mortality was 309 and 165, respectively, or 4 to 7 times lower [135]. Researchers wondered why. Probably, among other causes, the answer is in the latitude.

I learned about the CVD and latitude connection from Zoë Harcombe who tested the Keys' correlation between cholesterol and coronary heart disease in seven countries. Keys came up with the coefficient of linear correlation of 0.72 [136]. While looking at the Keys' original data, Harcombe noticed that the further north in Europe the country was located, the higher was the death rate. She determined the latitude of the Keys' seven countries and came up with a 0.93 coefficient of correlation [137, p.106; 138].

So, taking latitude as a risk factor for coronary heart disease, she could predict heart disease with higher accuracy than did Keys with his cholesterol. Although correlation reflects only the association between two parameters, not causation as she stressed, the casual factor could be vitamin D synthesis in our skin exposed to the sun.

Other than vitamin D, in colder climates, in order to maintain our body temperature, we need to produce more energy. Mitochondria, an energy generator unit in each of our cells, which burns glucose and fat, produces both energy for all body functions and heat. Just to warm up the cold air that we inhale requires additional heat to be produced by the body.

In the process of burning food for calories, free radicals are generated in mitochondria, which damage its DNA and fatty acids that compose the walls of mitochondria. The more calories we burn, the more metabolic waste we create, and the more damage is imposed on the mitochondria itself which accelerates its aging and a loss of efficiency both in energy production and self-maintenance and repair.

Exposed to cold, our blood vessels and skin capillaries shrink, which impairs microcirculation in our limbs. A study in Sweden demonstrated that the number of heart attacks in winter goes up [139]. There were also reports that shoveling after snowfall puts elderly folks, especially those with cardiovascular disease, into physical exertion that triggers heart attacks [140]. Being exposed to an extreme cold, some unfortunate people even lose their feet or hands due to frost bite, leading to and amputation, which would never happen in tropical climates.

Another challenge of living in cold areas is an increase of omega-3 in foods that, due to their high Peroxidability Index, are always oxidized, rancid, aged, and stale. Omega-3 being liquid at near-freezing temperatures insures germination of seeds and grains in the cold spring both in the northern regions and high in the mountains.

Rice, which is grown in warm areas, has the lowest omega-3 content of 44 mg (brown rice) and 31 mg (white rice) in 100 g of the grain. Buckwheat, oats and rye grown in colder areas (Canada and Russia) have omega-3 level of 78 mg, 111 mg and 157 mg, respectively. Two grains that come from high altitudes in the mountains of South America, namely quinoa and chia (mila) are high in omega-3.

Quinoa contains 307 mg and chia, which is reputed as the wonder grain of ancient Aztecs, has 17,552 mg, the second highest (after flaxseeds) level of all grains [141].

Among seeds and nuts, coconuts growing in the tropics do not have omega-3 at all, almonds and Brazil nuts that grow in warm areas have 6 mg and 18 mg, respectively. Rapeseeds (source of rapeseed or canola oil) contain 40-45% oil [142] of which omega-3 comprises 9.4-10.4% [143]. The omega-3 content in rapeseeds, hemp seeds, and flaxseeds cultivated in cold Canada and Russia are much higher, 421 mg, 7,143 mg, and 22,813 mg in 100 g of seeds, respectively [141].

The same picture is with fish, warm water fish such as tuna, cod or snapper are low in omega-3, 243 mg, 195 mg, and 380 mg, respectively and cold water salmon (2,018 mg) [144] and sardines (1,480 mg) [145] in 100 grams of fish are much higher. When we consume these high omega-3 foods, we expose our tissues and organs to toxic lipid peroxidation aldehydes such as HNE and MDA which cause inflammation, promote the development of atherosclerosis and lead to heart attacks and strokes.

To test the idea if there is a link between mortality and latitude, I analyzed the all-cause mortality [146] of the 25 high-income countries [147]. The latitude for each country can be easily found on the Internet. The relationship between all-cause mortality and latitude is shown in Figure 1.

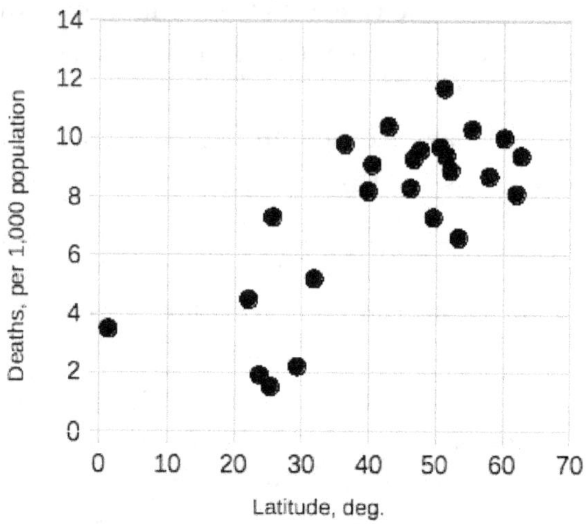

Figure 1. All-Cause Deaths versus Latitude: for 25 Countries

DESPITE THE NOTICEABLE scatter of the dots, one can see an evident upward trend in the number of deaths that go up hand-in-hand with increasing latitude. The left-most dot represents Singapore (1.3°N latitude, 3.5 deaths per 1,000 population), the right-most dot-Sweden (62.7°N latitude, 9.4 deaths), the uppermost dot-Germany (51.2°N latitude, 11.7 deaths), and the lower-most dot-Qatar (25.3°N latitude, 1.5 deaths).

The standard Pearson correlation coefficient for this graph is 0.73, which is higher than the 0.63 value "indicating a positive association" between two parameters, not due to random chance [148]. This is an association, not causation, but it indicates that probably latitude can be considered as an additional risk factor for all-cause mortality.

The link between cardiovascular disease CVD mortality and latitude also seems to be the case, although the correlation is lower. The above-discussed study in Russia [135] showed a stark predominance of the CVD mortality in northern over the southern regions, but a similar comparison for Alaska (4.7 %) and Hawaii (3.7 %) in the USA did not reveal a big difference [161]. Probably, in the USA other factors than latitude play major role.

The CVD mortality data, both for men and women [162], is plotted against latitude of 25 high-income countries (Figure 2).

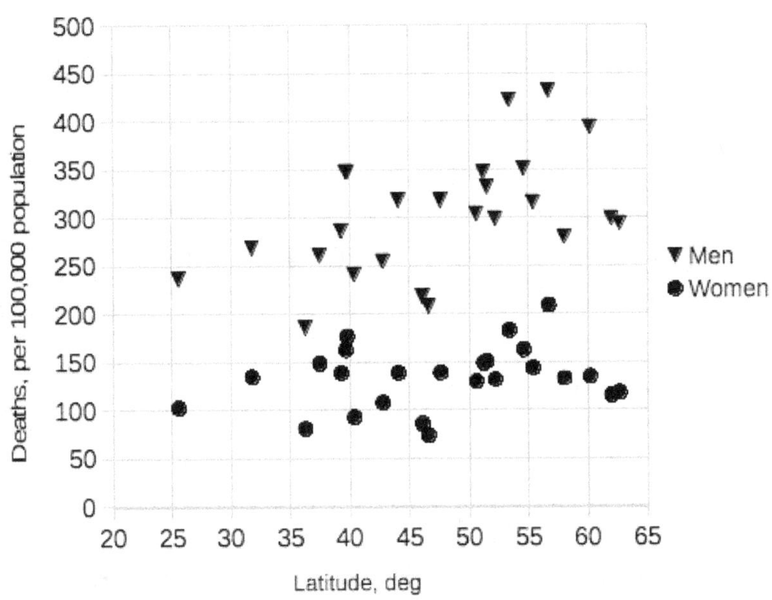

FIGURE 2. CVD Deaths vs. Latitude for 25 Countries

THE SCATTER IS noticeable again and the correlation coefficient for men is 0.50 (>0.43) and for women it is a mere 0.25 (<0.43). Using 0.43 as criteria of the association significance, we can say that only men but not women fall under the spell of latitude. With their higher body fat content, women are less vulnerable to the adverse effects of cold climates than men, as Figure 2 shows. So, we can say that women are "immune" to latitude, an additional risk factor for heart disease.

This graph also demonstrates that men in every country have nearly double the CVD mortality rates than women.

The difference between male and female mortality from CVD disease goes up with increasing latitude (Figure 3).

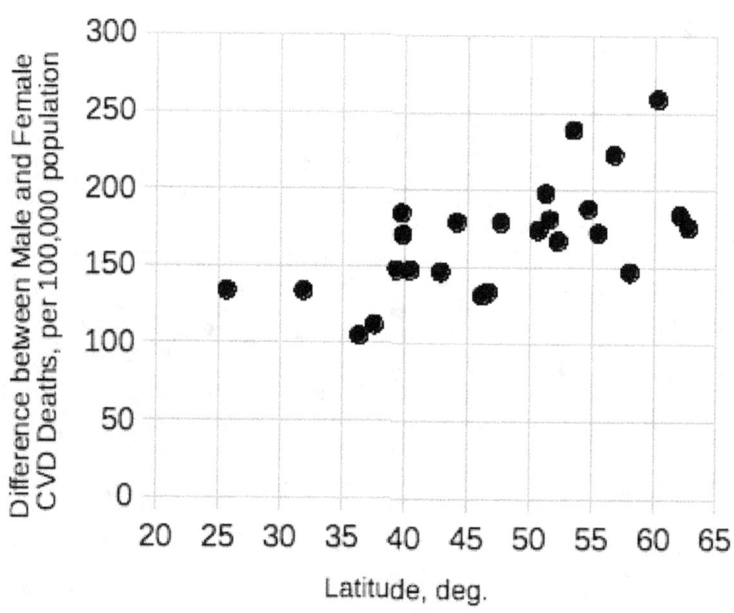

FIGURE 3. Difference between Annual Male and Female CVD Deaths vs. Latitude for 25 Countries

THE CORRELATION COEFFICIENT for this plot is 0.64 (>0.43), even higher than 0.50 for men in Figure 2, indicating that men's heart easily gives up when it is cold. Definitely, men are no match to women in surviving the CVD odds.

In every country in which they live, women enjoy 5 to 6 years longer life than men [146]. In the game of life, women undoubtedly are winners and men are humanity's lemons.

4

HOW OUR HEART AND CIRCULATION FUNCTIONS:

Since men have double the CVD mortality rates compared to women, it is important for them to acquire more knowledge about the heart, circulation, heart disease, and how to avoid it. Conventional wisdom maintains that heart disease is caused by atherosclerosis, a narrowing and hardening of the coronary arteries. Let's take a closer look at how atherosclerosis develops. At the beginning of atherosclerosis, the endothelial cells lining the arterial wall are injured. The multiple causes of endothelial injury include advancing age [151], biological, e.g. bacterial infection by microorganisms [152, p.171], hemodynamic, e.g. shear stress on the vessel wall induced by the blood flow [153], and chemical, e.g. smoking, elevated C-reactive protein, homocysteine, oxidized LDL cholesterol and circulating endotoxins [154], hypertension, diabetes [9, p.981], and others. "Vegetable oils, partially hydrogenated fats, and fried foods are responsible for the persistently high rate of heart disease" [154].

The PUFA-derived endotoxins such as HNE, HHE and MDA circulating in the blood, oxidize LDL cholesterol, irritate the lining of blood vessels and cause their inflammation. The inflamed endothelium cells fail to produce "normal amounts of antithrombotic and vasodilating cytokines" [9, p.981].

Following the activation of endothelial inflammation, the reactive oxygen species generated in the adventitia (outer layer of the arterial wall) oxidize LDL cholesterol. The immune system response "triggers expression of adhesion molecules (selectins and integrines) in the arterial endothelium, stimulating adhesion of monocytes to endothelium" [155, p.246].

The accumulation and oxidation of LDL in the developing lesion and induction of monocytes is followed by their infiltration into the arterial intima (inner layer of the arterial wall) through the junctions between endothelial cells. Once inside the arterial intima, monocytes differentiate into macrophages that engulf oxidized LDL becoming foam cells. "The macrophage foam cells generate ROS, produce tumor necrosis factor-α (TNF-α) and interleukin-1 (IL-1), and matrix metallo-proteinase 9 (MMP-9) that promote atherosclerosis..." [155, p.246].

Foam cells accumulated in large amounts form a lesion known as a fatty streak. "These lesions can be found in the walls of the arteries of most people, even young children. Once formed, fatty streaks produce more toxic oxygen radicals and cause immunologic and inflammatory changes, resulting in progressive damage to the vessel wall" [9, p.981].

The fibrous plaque, containing smooth muscle cells, collagen, cellular waste products, and oxidized LDL, accumulated in the lipid pool, forms the core of the plaque [156, p.1073]; progressive deposition of fibrin and calcium contribute over decades to the narrowing (stenosis) of the artery and eventually to complete obstruction of the artery and a "heart attack," aka myocardial infarction. Interestingly, slowly progressive coronary artery disease is not the main cause of a myocardial infarction. Actually, only one in eight heart attacks is attributed to chronic, slowly progressing stenosis as depicted by Dr. Caldwell B. Esselstyn, Jr. in his book, *Prevent and Reverse Heart Disease*: three drawings show a gradual build-up of a plaque inside the coronary artery leading to almost complete closing of the lumen (vessel inner channel).

However, most heart attacks originate in arteries that harbor blockages with less than 50% stenosis. How is this possible? It turns out that developing plaques, that do not impair downstream blood flow and hence cause no symptoms, can become unstable and "rupture" causing platelet adherence to the fissures which then initiate "the coagulation cascade and result in rapid thrombus formation with complete vessel occlusion causing tissue ischemia and infarction" [9, p.984].

The thrombus formed on the top of the fibrous plaque, is unstable and can be dislodged by the blood flow current. It can block the artery and stop the blood flow downstream. If the thrombus originates in the carotid artery it can lead to a stroke. If the thrombus originates in the aorta, it can lodge in distally and cause infarction of the abdominal vessels, kidney vessels and even leg arteries (blue toe syndrome).

Preventing conventional heart attacks means preventing the plaque from slowly closing the artery and also, more importantly, preventing the non-obstructive plaque from "sudden rupture." If the blood flow to the heart muscle diminishes or stops, the heart muscle cannot function at optimum parameters, hence the development of "heart failure." There are also other factors contributing to the development of "heart failure."

In conventional medicine, it is widely accepted that the heart is a pump. The *Taber's Cyclopedic Medical Dictionary* defines the heart as "A hollow, muscular organ, the pump of the circulatory system" [158, p.1018]. The *Pathophysiology* describes the function of circulation as a delivery system of oxygen and nutrients to organs and tissues and removal of waste products. Furthermore, "Delivery and removal are achieved by an extreme array of tubing—the blood and lymphatic vessels—connected to a pump—the heart" [156, p.1017]. Albert F. Blaisdell, MD, in his book, *Our Bodies and How We Live*, published in 1902, explains how the blood supply to organs and tissues is furnished by "some special machinery" of which, "... there is in the chest a powerful forcing-pump, called the heart" [159, p.126].

This mechanistic view of the heart as a pump among cardiologists continued for nearly four centuries since William Harvey (1578-1657), a British physician introduced it in 1628 [160, p.7]. Contrary to the popular belief that the "heart is a pump" notion, some researchers have denied it. In the 1995 article, *The heart is not a pump: A refutation of the pressure propulsion premise of heart function*, Ralph Marinelli, et al. argue "that the heart was not a pump forcing inert blood to move with pressure but that the blood was propelled with its own biological momentum, as can be seen in the embryo, and boosts itself with "induced" momenta from the heart" [161]. The authors further write that blood moves through the vessels autonomously in swirling, vortex streams, as in whirlpools or tornadoes. In contrast, conventional medicine views blood moving under the pressure created by the pumping heart in a laminar flow of concentric layers or turbulent flow when blood vessels branch or blood flow is obstructed, e.g., by the plaque [156, p.1043].

Pointing out an impossibility for the heart, which weighs about 300 grams, to push five liters of blood through all the 75,000 miles of capillaries, which are thinner than the size of the red blood cell, authors of the article note, "Also, the concept of a centralized pressure source (the heart) generating excessive pressure at its source, so that sufficient pressure remains at the remote capillaries, is not an elegant one" [161]. Nicely put but one can hear their mind crying out, "What a strange a concept!"

What is a pump? Dictionaries give many definitions, but the most common is: "A force-creating instrument that causes fluids to move." This definition confines the heart to its only ejecting, pressure-producing action. The more appropriate definition, in my view, comes from *Webster's Deluxe Unabridged Dictionary* which defines pump as, "any of various machines that force a liquid or gas into, or draw it out of, something, as by suction or pressure" [162, p.1461].

The double-action property of a pump in this definition reflects the ejecting and sucking actions of all four chambers of the heart during their contractions and relaxations. Although the term 'relaxation' is widely used, it does not reflect of what is happening in all four chapters of the heart. For instance, the pressure inside left ventricle drops to almost zero at the end of the cardiac cycle [163, p.22]. Therefore, the term 'collapse' seems to be more appropriate.

The authors of the article explain the commonly measured blood pressure, which is the pressure on the artery walls, as the pressure on the object which interrupts the flow of blood moving with momentum.

As a result of obstruction of blood flow, "...the velocity decreases while the pressure of a certain magnitude appears." Rudolf Steiner, scientist and philosopher, pointed out "that the pressure is not the cause of blood flow but the result of it" [164].

The most important factors influencing blood flow, according to the conventional medicine, are blood pressure and the resistance of blood vessels [156, p.1042]. Other factors include blood velocity, its viscosity (thickness), laminar or turbulent flow, and blood vessel compliance, which is the opposite of stiffness that can be caused by aging or arteriosclerosis [156, p.1043]. Various parameters of blood vessels involved in the circulation are shown in Table 15-7.

Table 15-7. Parameters of Blood Vessels

Blood Vessel	Diameter, mm	Length, mm	Total Cross Section, mm^2	Resistance, Pa*s/ml	Blood Velocity, cm/sec		Reynolds Number
Aorta	20	500	250	0.008	50	48	3,400
Arteries	4	500	3,000	2.3	10-40	45	500
Arterioles	0.05	10	4,000	99.1	20	5	0.7
Capillaries	0.008	1	250,000	12.1	0.03	0.1	0.002
Venules	0.02	2	25,000	44.1	0.3	0.2	0.01
Veins	5	25	8,000	0.03	0.3-5	10	140
Vena Cava	30	500	800	0.0008	5-20	38	3,300
Source	[227]	[227]	[227]	[227]	[227]	[382]	[382]

BLOOD PRESSURE, both systolic and diastolic, resistance, and blood velocity are plotted in Figure 4 along the route of blood flow starting from the heart's aorta, then through arteries, arterioles, capillaries, venules, veins and eventually returning to the heart via the venae cavae. Blood pressure gradually decreases from e.g., 120/82 mm Hg at the exit of the heart to 2 mm Hg at the vena cava. The curves for systolic and diastolic pressures meet at the beginning of the capillaries at 61 mm Hg and after this point the distinction between systolic and diastolic pressures disappears [158, p.288].

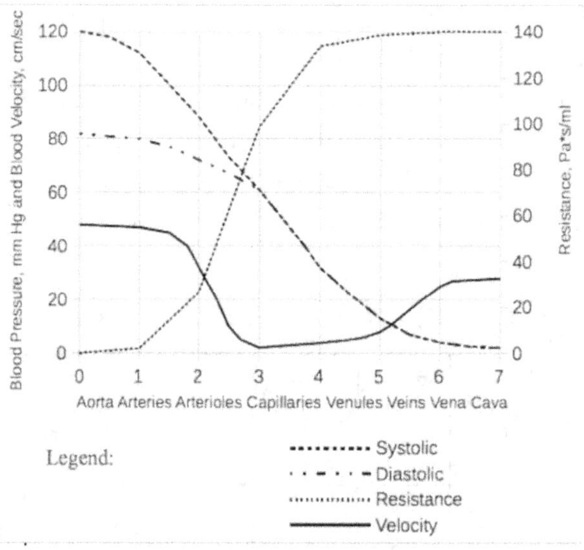

Figure 4. Changes of Blood Pressure, Resistance, and Velocity in Blood Vessels

RESISTANCE (R), which is opposition to the flow of liquid under pressure through the vessel, according to Poiseuille's law, is proportional to the difference (ΔP) between pressures at the inflow (P1) and outflow (P2) ends of the vessel and inversely proportional to liquid flow (Q).

Liquid flow (Q) is a volume of liquid, e.g., in cm^3 moving through the vessel in a unit of time, e.g., in 1 sec. Jean Léonard Marie Poiseuille (1797-1869), a French physicist and physiologist developed an equation for non-turbulent blood flow in a tube in 1838 [165]. According to the Poiseuille's formula, $\mathbf{R = 8\eta l/\pi\ r^4}$, resistance (R) to flow through a single vessel is directly related to the liquid viscosity (η), length of the vessel (l), and inversely related to the fourth power of the vessel's radius (r^4). It is evident from the Poiseuille's formula that the caliber of the vessel's lumen expressed as its radius (r) in the 4th power is the most important factor determining resistance to blood flow.

Being the lowest in the aorta, resistance increases slightly in the arteries and sharply in the arterioles, and then continues to rise in the capillaries. In the capillaries, with their infinitesimally small lumen of 0.008 mm [158, p.358], or even 0.002-0.003 mm [166], one would expect resistance to increase in a sky-rocketing manner, but it does not, as the resistance curve in Figure 4 shows. Beyond the capillary bed, resistance continues to build in the venules, veins, and venae cavae but in a less dramatic fashion.

Resistance (R) to blood flow in the Poiseuille's formula is directly proportional to the vessel's length (l) and blood viscosity (η). Blood viscosity is determined by its hematocrit (volume of blood occupied by blood cells), plasma viscosity, the tendency of red blood cells to form aggregates, and their deformability [167]. A value of blood viscosity measured by a viscosimeter is 5 mPa*s, or 5 times greater than that of water [168]. Total peripheral blood vessel resistance (R) is estimated as 140 Pa*s/ml and the contribution of each circulation portion is: aorta and arteries-19%, arterioles-50%, capillaries-25%, all veins-4%, and metarterioles plus thoroughfare channels-3% [168].

Hobbie, R. K. and Roth, B. J. in their book, *Intermediate Physics for Medicine and Biology*, give another example of the total resistance (R) obtained from the formula, $R = \Delta P/Q$. They use the average pressure ΔP, e.g. 100 mm Hg and the average blood flow (Q) from the heart, which is the stroke volume determined as the volume of blood ejected in each beat, e.g. 60 ml/beat, multiplied by the number of beats per minute, e.g. 80 beat/min to obtain a cardiac output of 4800 ml/min. They come up with the value of $R = 1.66*10^8 \, Pa \, m^{-3} \, s$ [163, p.21].

In another example, the average cardiac output in a normal resting adult is 5 L/min [9, p.951] which results in $R = 1.60*10^8 \, Pa \, m^{-3} \, s$. Since 1 m^3 of fluid is equal to 10^6 ml, we obtain R = 166 Pa*s/ml and R = 160 Pa*s/ml for both calculations, which are close enough to the indicated above value of 140 Pa*s/ml [168].

It is tempting to determine resistance (Rc) to blood flow in a single blood vessel including capillary using Poiseuille's formula and compare those with the total resistance (R) of the systemic circulation. As for the value of the blood viscosity in the capillary, we need to consider the notion that "In blood vessels of less than 100 μm radius, the apparent viscosity decreases with tube radius" [163, p.23].

On the other hand, the existence on the interior surfaces of the capillaries of a thin layer of "macromolecules bound or absorbed to the endothelium," called glycocalyx, increases flow resistance and the "presence of a 1/2-micron-thick glycocalyx in a 5-micron capillary results in a threefold increase in resistance and a reduction in the capillary tube hematocrit of more than 30% compared with the corresponding values in a 5-micron smooth-walled tube" [169].

In the capillaries of 8 microns in diameter, red blood cells that are about of the same size move in a single file, and each cell is surrounded by plasma, which also separates cells from the capillary wall. Therefore, it seems reasonable to assume the capillary blood viscosity as that of plasma viscosity (η), which is estimated to be equal to $\eta = 1.5*10^{-3}$ Pa s [170]. As compared with that of water, $0.692*10^{-3}$ N m^{-2} s [163, p.90], of the same temperature of 37 °C, the capillary plasma viscosity is 2.17 times larger, although blood viscosity can be 5 times greater than that of water [168]. For an average capillary diameter 0.008 mm and length 1 mm [163, p.21], Rc = $1.49*10^8$ x Pa s/ml. The values of (R) for a single capillary and other single blood vessels are shown in Table 15-7.

It appears that the resistance (Rc) to blood flow in a single capillary is 10^8 or **100 million times** larger than that of the whole body systemic circulation ($1.66*10^8$ Pa m^{-3} s [163, p.21]). Even the resistance of a single arteriole or venule is about **one million times** more than the whole body systemic resistance.

The above value of Rc is enormous, but before you would probably think that it is unreasonable to apply the Poiseuille equation to blood flow in the capillaries because of their very small size and the 4th power of their radius, consider this.

Hobbit and Roth give an example of using the Poiseuille equation to determine a flow (i) of a liquid moving through the pore "in the basement membrane of the glomerulus of the kidney." The pore size is 5 nm (nanometer, one-thousandth of the micron), the length is 50 nm, the pressure gradient is ΔP = 15.4 mm Hg, and the liquid viscosity (η) is $1.4*10^{-3}$kg m^{-1} s^{-1}. The result of their calculation is: i = $7.2*10^{-21}$ m^3 s^{-1} [163, p.17]. Hobbie and Roth stop here without explaining what it actually means, but I will try to explain it to you. If we convert cubic meters in their example into cubic millimeters, we obtain i = $7.2*10^{-12}$ mm^3 s^{-1}.

The droplets of fog or mist in a cloud are 10-15 microns in size and the volume of the 10 micron droplet is $5.24*10^{-7}$ mm^3. It means that the liquid amount equal to **one 0.14 millionth** of the mist droplet will pass in their example through that pore per second. It is so infinitesimally small that it begs a question if it is tenable to use the Poiseuille equation in this case. If it is, then our calculation for a much larger (one thousand times) capillary resistance seems to be justified.

Because resistance (R) is affected the most by both vessel's lumen and the "number of vessels recruited" [158, p.2007], during the exercise more capillaries will become active and resistance will be even greater. What is the number of capillaries? If we assume the mean diameter of one capillary of being 0.008 mm, then in their total cross section area of 250,000 mm^2 [102] the number of capillaries will be 4,976,114,649, or close to 5 billion capillaries.

The common explanation in the physiology books [9] and [102] that resistance of the capillary bed is not that great involves a notion that capillaries are arranged in both series and in parallel. If they are connected in the series, than total resistance is a sum of individual resistances: $.R_1 + R_2 + R_3 + ...$ In the branching vessels, if they are connected to the feeding vessel in parallel, their total resistance is $1/R_1 + 1/R_2 + 1/R_3 + ...$ Then, the total resistance is smaller than that of a single vessel.

Hobbie and Roth maintain that "For the most part, the capillaries are arranged in parallel. Even though the resistance of an individual capillary is large because of its small radius (Eq. 1.58), the resistance of the capillaries as a whole is relatively small because there are so many of them" [163, p.20-21]. 'For the most part...' says a lot, but unfortunately does not specify how many of the capillaries are arranged in parallel or in series. If only two capillaries of five plus billion are arranged in series, the total resistance would be astronomical, as the above calculation example for a single capillary showed.

The above calculation has limitations because the blood viscosity η = 1.5 mPa*s is assumed to be the same for different blood vessels. As a non-Newtonian fluid, blood (a suspension) has varying viscosity (η) depending on its velocity or shear strength: viscosity is the lowest at 5 mPa*s at the exit from the heart where blood moves the fastest, increases to 10 mPa*s in the arteries and becomes as great as 800 mPa*s in the capillary bed where its speed is the slowest [168]. Because of that, the total resistance of the capillary bed would be beyond any wild imagination.

Now, if we look at the blood velocity curve in Figure 4, we can see that the blood velocity decreases from 48 cm/sec at the heart exit to the lowest level of 0.03 cm/sec [106] at the beginning of the capillaries, rises to 2 cm/sec at their end (within only 0.5-1 mm of their length), and further increases while passing venules, veins, and venae cavae to 38 cm/sec at the heart door [171].

With decreasing vessel diameter, the blood velocity decreases, the pressure continue to drop and the total resistance should skyrocket (Figure 4). Under these conditions, the blood flow in capillaries should stop but instead, the speed of blood movement in capillaries and past the capillary bed is increases progressively reaching the right atrium. With only 2 mm Hg (or 1.7%) of blood pressure left, and huge resistance to blood flow encountered, how is this possible?

The conventional explanation relates the increase in blood velocity to the decrease of the total cross-sectional area of vessels past the capillary bed, stating that, "When capillaries merge into venules and venules merge into veins, the total cross-sectional area decreases, causing flow rate to increase" [156, Fig.32.24, p.1042].

A bit earlier, on the same page we read, "The most important factors that influence blood flow are pressure and resistance, followed by velocity, turbulent versus laminar flow, and compliance" [156, p.1042]. The velocity (v) is directly proportional to the volume blood flow (Q) in a vessel and inversely proportional to the vessel's cross-sectional area (S). In its turn, blood flow (Q) is related to the pressure gradient (ΔP) and resistance (R). For a bundle (N) of small parallel tubes, G. B. Thurston has modified the Poiseuille's equation for a pressure-to-flow relationship [172].

In the above conventional explanation, of three factors determining blood flow rate (v) in the arteries, capillaries, and veins, two factors, namely (ΔP) and (R) seem to be suddenly lost and what remains is only (S), the "total cross-sectional area." It does not look tenable at all. Further, the explanation goes on stating, "Because resistance reaches a maximal level in the arteries, they are sometimes called the "stop-cocks" of the vascular system" [9, p.960].

This is not true. As one can see from Table 15-7, the contribution of the aorta and arteries to the total resistance is only 19%, and it is much lower than in arterioles (51%) and capillaries (25%). Thus, in terms of resistance, arterioles and capillaries are much more "stop-cocks" than arteries. Further on, "Many capillaries arise from each arteriole so that the total cross-sectional area of the capillary bed is very large and resistance is low, despite the fact that the cross-sectional area of each capillary is less (which normally increases resistance) than that of each arteriole" [9, p.960].

It is not that simple, although the resistance of the capillary bed is half of that in the arterioles (25% versus 51% in Table 15-7), it is governed by different factors specific to capillaries, e.g. decreased blood viscosity, changing chemical factors, electrical charge, etc., discussed below.

And more, "As a result, blood flow becomes quite slow in the capillaries, analogous to water flow in a river. A narrow river whose bed widens flows more slowly through the wide section than through the narrow section" [9, p.960]. A similar comparison with the water flowing in "a swift river emptying into a large lake" where its speed decreases "until it becomes almost imperceptible" is found in the *Human Anatomy & Physiology* book [173, p.734].

A comparison of blood flowing in the multiple closed tube-like blood vessels to the water flowing in the river is grossly inappropriate because the river is one and blood vessels are counted in millions (arterioles and venules) and billions (capillaries). Also, the river is not a closed tube fully filled (no air space) with the flowing liquid in it. It seems that conventional cardiology cannot explain the slow blood flow in the capillaries other than by their increased total cross-sectional area.

Robert C. Little, MD, the physiology professor and William C. Little, MD, the cardiology associate professor, in their book, *Physiology of the Heart and Circulation*, state, "In the capillaries, the total cross-sectional area increases 700 to 800 times, and the vascular stream widens into a large lake. Due to the reciprocal relationship described earlier between velocity and total cross-sectional area, the capillary flow becomes very slow" [174, p.228].

The comparison of blood circulation with water flowing in the river is not that uncommon and even critical minds fall into this trap. Thomas Cowan, MD, a cardiologist who challenged the widely accepted "heart is a pump" dogma, did a similar comparison too. He asserts, "If you examine the relative velocity of the blood at various stages of the circulation, you'll see that the blood moves the fastest in the large arteries and veins, where it is forced into comparatively fewer channels, and the blood moves the slowest in the capillaries, because there are so many of them" [160, p.9].

Cowan doesn't mention pressure, resistance, and the infinitesimal size of the capillaries; he emphasizes just the number of vessels. Then he continues, "This is similar to how water moves in a river. It is fastest when the river is narrow, slower when it flows out into tributaries and slowest when it flows out into a wetland area" [160, p.9]. Blood flow through billions of tubular capillaries and water moving in the "wetland area" is regarded as "similar." Actually, the 250,000 mm^2 total cross-sectional area of the capillary bed is equal to a tube of 443 mm or 0.443 m in diameter or 18 times larger than that of the aorta.

With this logic, blood in capillaries must move much slower than in the aorta, and it does but for a completely different reason. Each capillary, that is only one-tenth the thickness of a human hair (40-120 microns), creates a tremendous resistance to blood flow. The capillary bed, distributed in all organs and tissues of the body, is composed of 5+ billion these tiny tubes. Blood moves through each of them, not through the "total cross-sectional area" where the borders of individual vessels are deemed not to exist. Therefore, indication of the total cross-sectional area as a determining factor of blood velocity in the capillaries is absolutely irrelevant. This explanation does not hold even a drop of water, leave the drop of blood alone.

This "blood vessels-river" comparison sounds to me less than elegant, if not plainly wrong. Again, blood flows the slowest (actually nearly stops) in the capillaries because of the much-decreased pressure gradient and their enormous resistance, but not their total cross-sectional area. Dr. Robert C. Atkins would call that kind of logic the cognitive dissonance, I guess. The Medical dictionary defines "cognitive dissonance" as "Incongruity of thought, philosophy, or action" [158, p.674]. Incongruous means out of place, absurd.

5

BLOOD FLOW IN CAPILLARIES

So, what moves the blood through capillaries then and even accelerates a flow rate from their arterioles end to the venules end? The answer is surprisingly simple: capillaries themselves and the processes occurring in them. Capillaries being infinitely small and seen only under microscope nevertheless have a complex structure. In a lengthwise section, a capillary contains six layers [175].

On the outside of the capillary wall built by the endothelial cells is a basement membrane. It is separated from endothelial cells by the endothelial space. On the inside of endothelial cells is an endothelial fibrin film that borders a layer of relatively immobile plasma and finally there is a mobile plasma at the vessel's center [176].

Contractions of capillaries that promote blood flow are enhanced by the nerve cells attached to them. "The capillaries, small vessel arteries, and veins are provided with nerve fibers which evidently offer one possibility for neurogenous impulses of contraction" [177, p.141]. Another possibility is related to the pericytes, the cells of ellipsoidal shape which are adjacent to the outside of capillary walls and scattered along the capillaries. "Pericytes are described as involved in the mechanism of contraction of arterioles, venules and capillaries" [177, p.137].

Capillaries are so small that red blood cells being larger in diameter must bend, elongate or acquire a bullet form to be able to squeeze through them moving in a single file [9, p.956, micrograph 500 x]. Normally having a form of biconcave discoid, red blood cells (erythrocytes) in the tight capillaries can acquire a bell shape moving forward with its protruding end, somewhat resembling a jellyfish moving in the water with its train behind its main body. In the bell shape, the surface area of erythrocyte is 10% larger [168]. Blood cells do not touch capillary walls but are separated from them with a thin layer (boundary zone) of plasma, which is 0.0005 to 0.0010 mm thick [168].

Water that comprises 91.5% of plasma [158, p.1800] while moving in the hydrophilic (water-loving) blood vessels forms an "exclusion zone" of structured water [178]. The 'layer" of this structured water is only three or four molecules thick but it has different properties than ordinary "bulk" water: free of toxins, solutes, and other substances (hence "exclusion"), higher density and viscosity, negative electrical charge, and altered pH values [160, p.12-14].

In the process of water structuring, separation of charges takes place: structured water becomes infused with the free electrons having a negative charge while the bulk water becomes enriched with protons that are positively charged. This ionization of water brings about astounding repercussions—the bulk water begins to move since positively charged ions repel each other.

The blood in the capillaries moves in the forward direction from arterioles to venues because it is acted upon by the "vis a tergo" force (force from behind) which comes with each left ventricle contraction as a "pressure wave" with the speed of sound, as was established by the Russian scientist, N. E. Zhukovsky [168].

The very slow flow of blood through capillaries ensures a proper discharge of oxygen from erythrocytes and nutrients from blood plasma into the interstitial liquid surrounding capillaries and collection of the carbon dioxide and end products of cell metabolism such as uric acid, urea, lactic acid, and ammonia.

The filtration of water from the capillary into the surrounding interstitial fluid and its reabsorption back into the capillary is determined by the interactions of the capillary hydrostatic pressure HP and the capillary colloid osmotic pressure OP opposing it. The osmotic pressure OP is created by the water-attracting plasma proteins (primarily albumin) in the capillary blood. At the arterial end of the capillary bed, HP is higher than OP, which is driving water out of the capillary. On the venous end of the capillary bed, the OP becomes dominant, and the water is drawn back to the capillary bed [173, p.739-740].

In the tight capillaries, red blood cells move in a single file and the blood hematocrit is much lower, e.g., ~15% in resting muscle as compared to ~45% in muscles during exercise or in larger blood vessels [170]. This loss of water at the arterial end of the capillary bed and its influx towards the venous end affects hematocrit in a way that it is somewhat increased above its capillary ~15% and then decreased with more watery plasma. Accordingly, the capillary blood viscosity becomes progressively lower along the capillaries towards their venous end.

The end products of cellular metabolism such as carbon dioxide CO_2 and lactic acid (from oxidation of glucose and fatty acids), urea, uric acid, ammonia, from amino acids metabolized predominantly in the liver and some in the skeletal muscles are released from cells into interstitial fluid and further infused into capillary blood.

In the capillary blood, carbon dioxide CO_2 dissolves in plasma and by the action of the carbonic anhydrase enzyme forms carbonic acid. Some CO_2 binds to hemoglobin of the erythrocytes to form a compound called carbaminohemoglobin. The acidity of carbonic acid forces oxygen bound to hemoglobin (oxyhemoglobin) of red blood cells into the interstitial fluid. In the capillaries of the lung alveoli, the reverse exchange of carbon dioxide and oxygen takes place [179, p.36].

Because of their infinitesimal and ever-changing lumen, and the extreme complexity of the processes occurring in capillaries in different tissues and organs, the ordinary laws of fluid dynamics including the Poiseuille's law can hardly be applied to them [180].

The capillaries are considered "largely independent of systemic factors" dealing with the physical factors. Chemical metabolic factors, though, such as potassium and hydrogen ions, adenosine, lactic acid, prostaglandins, released from cells and nitric oxide NO produced by their endothelial cells may play a significant role in blood flow through them [160, p.734-35]. The fact remains that the speed of blood cell flow in the capillaries at their arterioles end of 0.3 mm/sec increases to 20 mm/sec at the venules end. This is despite a drop of pressure and increasing resistance. Why?

Is it chemical substances, e.g., metabolic products of the capillary exchange entering capillaries? There are indications that urine which contains urea and uric acid "improves blood flow and lymph circulation" [181, p.139]. The capillary action, water "exclusion zone," electrical charges, metabolic factors and something else that is not discovered yet may hold a key to the capillary mystery.

We often pretend that we already know, but it turns out we don't. Mother Nature hasn't revealed to us yet all the secrets of Her creation. Science makes discoveries every day, and maybe we will better understand how capillaries function in the future. As Daniel J. Boorstin, the National Librarian of Congress, pointed out in 1983, "The greatest impediment to scientific progress is not ignorance but the illusion of knowledge" [182].

The capillary action (capillary effect), which is widely present in nature, allows, for instance, sap to reach the top of 300-foot trees pulling it up from the roots. Curiously, in a Wikipedia's *Capillary Action* article, the capillary action is mentioned taking place in small animals such as the wharf roach *Ligia exotica* and an agamid lizard *Moloch horridus*is living in Australia that can absorb water by capillary-like structures in their legs (the former) and skin (the latter). In humans, it is observed in the so-called lacrimal ducts which drain tear liquid that is constantly produced to lubricate our eyes [183].

Whether the "capillary action" phenomenon is applicable to animal and human blood circulation or not remains controversial. On one hand, physiologist Joseph Ahrens, Ph.D., from University of Florida denies it on the grounds that there is no adhesion of plasma and blood cells to vessel walls and no attraction (cohesion) in the blood itself. He further asserts. "We have a frictionless system..." [184].

However, the "...presence of a thick endothelial surface layer (ESL)" that is attached to the small vessel walls was found to increase blood flow resistance in the rats study [185]. The same view is held by Kim Aaron, Ph.D., in fluid dynamics from Caltech, saying that, "Capillary action only occurs when there is a free surface (such as the air-water interface inside the capillary tube). The blood capillaries are like parallel resistors so the heart can pump blood through them all..." [184].

On the other hand, the cardiologist Cowan admits that kind of possibility. He emphasizes the existence of the "exclusion zone" of the electron-enriched structured water attached to the hydrophilic endothelial cells of the inside of capillary wall, which has an increased viscosity compared with the bulk water in the center of the capillary. The "exclusion zone" is negatively charged and the positively charged protons inside capillary repel each other and cause the blood flow [160, p.12-5].

Dr. August Krogh (1874-1949) of Denmark was awarded a Nobel Prize in Physiology or Medicine in 1920 for his research of a capillary microcirculation in skeletal muscles. Krogh emphasized the importance of capillaries stating, "All exchange between the blood and the organs, of nutrient materials and waste products, of oxygen and carbon dioxide, takes place through their walls. In them, the blood fulfills its real function. One could say that the whole circulatory machine exists for their sake" [166]. The capillary beds are the site where the nourishing broth produced by the digestive and pulmonary systems and delivered through the circulation system is fed to the cells and their excretions are taken away.

More than that, the capillaries' ability to enhance circulation itself has fascinated many researchers and doctors. Alexander S. Zalmanov, MD (1875-1964), a prominent Russian physician who served as a family doctor of Vladimir Lenin, a Russian Bolshevik leader, and worked with Krogh, called capillaries the "second heart." Cowan was thrilled with the capillary circulation to the extent that he called it "a perpetual motion machine" [160, p.15].

6

BLOOD FLOW IN VEINS

Past miraculous capillaries, the blood in the wider venules merging into even wider veins becomes subjected to the physical, more than physiological, factors again. Blood flow velocity increases by the action of a few factors. One of them is the contraction of skeletal muscles surrounding veins, especially in the legs in the standing position. The wavelike contractions propel blood flow upward and, because of its importance in the venous return to the heart, is termed "muscle pump." To prevent back flow of blood in veins, there are valves, especially in the lower limbs which also assist in venous return [9, p.958].

How great the "muscle pump" effect can be, shows the experiment conducted by Prof. A. I. Arinchin, a Corresponding member of the Academy of Sciences of Belarus. He has isolated the calf muscle of the body, connected it to an artificial circulation, and observed that muscle contractions were able to increase blood pressure to 200, 250 mm Hg and even more. The values that he measured largely exceeded 120 mm Hg, the pressure that the heart is pumping to in normal conditions [186]. Because of that, some call muscles a "peripheral heart."

Another factor that increases the venous blood flow is the action of the "vis a fronte" (in front) force. The diastolic pressure in the right atrium is negative, −2 mmHg [188] or -2 to-4 mmHg [168], and although hydrostatic blood pressure in vena cava is only 15 mmHg [187], the pressure gradient of 17-19 mmHg insures the venous return with increased speed. Negative diastolic pressure in the right atrium creates vacuum and the heart sucks in the blood. This sucking-ejecting double action signifies the heart as a sucking pump [188] and is in an agreement with the above-mentioned dictionary definition. The breathing cycle also contributes to the venous return: the negative intrathoracic pressure during inspiration "sucks" the venous blood into the thoracic cavity and hence towards the right atrium.

These factors combined speed up the venous blood in its return to the heart (up to 38 cm/s in Table 15-7) to the extent that its flow pattern turns from laminar (linear) to turbulent (non-laminar). This is reflected by the dimensionless Reynolds number N_R which is a function of the vessel's characteristic length (L) (equal to its diameter), velocity (v), density (ρ), and viscosity (η) of the fluid.

The greater the tube diameter, liquid velocity, and density and lower its viscosity, the larger N_R is. In a study of blood velocity in the ascending aorta of "15 persons (seven normal, seven with aortic valvular disease, one with prosthetic aortic valve)," the "turbulent flow occurred above the aortic valve during peak flow" in all participants. The peak Reynolds numbers in six normal subjects ranged from 5,700 to 8,900 and reached even 10,000 in one "normal individual with a high cardiac output" [169].

Hobbie & Roth state that, "When NR is greater than a few thousand, turbulence usually occurs" [163, p.22]. They list N_R values of 9400 for aorta, 1300 for arteries, **3000 for vena cava** in the systemic circulation (see Table 15-7), 7800 for arteries, and 2200 for veins of the pulmonary circulation [163, p.21].

They assert that, "Blood flows in laminar except in the ascending aorta and main pulmonary artery, where turbulence may occur during peak flow" [163, p.22]. Although the vena cava is not mentioned, its value of $N_R = 3000$ fits into their "a few thousand" distinction. It means that to some extent the turbulence flow may occur in the vena cava at the peak venous return by the sucking action of the right atrium as well.

More evidence that it can be the case comes from the data in the book of M. J. Rhodes indicating that the flow is considered turbulent at $N_R = 2000$ [183]. The same number of 2000 is found in [187, p.231]. Furthermore, Cowan maintains that, "The function of the heart is to create vortices." He calls the vertical vortex coming from the whole body circulation and horizontal vortex, from pulmonary circulation, "the cross of vortices" [160, p.40].

Next to consider is the fact that the **pulsatile** blood flow which is a characteristic to the aorta and big arteries and disappears in arterioles, capillaries, venules and veins, takes the stage again in vena cava. It was known already 50 years ago after a study in England on four healthy male volunteers aged 29 to 39.

The most amazing thing is that the volunteers were the authors of the study, medical doctors who experimented on themselves. "A small incision was made over an antecubital vein and the tip of the velocity transducer was introduced into it." The antecubital vein is located in front of the elbow. "The transducer was then passed under fluoroscopic control through the right atrium and into the Inferior Vena Cava (IVC)..." and positioned "...between the entry points of the hepatic and renal veins." The Blood flow velocity, ECG, atrial, and IVC pressures were recorded simultaneously in the resting and exercise experiments.

Authors who risked their lives for the sake of science were rewarded with great results: "The most striking observations were that the velocity of venous flow is remarkably **pulsatile**." They also found that in all four subjects the flow velocity waves are "similar to the right atrial pressure waves in their general features, but they are in anti-phase. That is, a rise in right atrial pressure generally accompanies a reduction in the centripetal flow velocity and vice versa" [153].

From their recordings (Figure 2 in [153]), for instance, I could determine that at rest with the drop of the atrial pressure from 5.9 mm Hg to -5.5 mm Hg (negative, vacuum pressure) the velocity increased from -4.6 cm/sec (back flow) to 26 cm/sec. With each pulse, the blood pressure in the inferior vena cava IVC oscillated between 0.04 mmHg to 0.50 mmHg. The peak flow velocities recorded in IVC of one subject were 45.3 cm/sec at rest and 146.7 cm/sec during exercise for 2.5 min. In the same subject, the lowest flow velocity at rest was 34.4 cm/sec [153].

To determine whether blood flow at these velocities was laminar or turbulent, we can use the Reynolds numbers calculator [190], which employs the following parameters: inner diameter of the vena cava L = 3 cm, blood density ρ = 1060 kg/m3 [191], whole blood viscosity at the body temperature of 98.5°F (37°C) η = 2.8 mPa*s [154].

For the above-indicated velocities, the corresponding Reynolds numbers N_R are 5140, 16645 and 3903. They all exceed 2000 which means that the blood flow was turbulent. The only case when N_R =1475 (smaller than 2000) occurred was for the lowest flow velocity of 13 cm/sec recorded in one of the subjects in this study [153]. However, the next to the lowest velocity, 18.9 cm/sec, obtained in yet another participant corresponded to N_R = 2144. It appears that the N_R = 2000 threshold for vena cava equals to the blood velocity of 17.6 cm/sec.

What these results mean is that the flow velocity was the greatest during the collapse and sucking action of the right atrium. If the only blood mover throughout the body is the **pulsatile** ejections of the heart's left ventricle, as the "heart is a pump" theory and practice holds, then how can **pulsatile** and **turbulent** flow in the venae cavae be explained?

Conventional cardiology acknowledges the presence of the negative right atrial pressure and its effects on venous return. Little & Little explaining the Guyton diagram, in which circulation is divided into heart-pump and peripheral circulation parts, assert, "If right atrial pressure falls below atmospheric, the negative pressure in the great veins causes them to collapse as they leave the chest. This obstruction prevents venous return from significantly increasing further if right atrial pressure falls to sub-atmospheric levels" [174, p.193-94]. On the Figure 7-20 [174, p.193], one can estimate that right atrial pressure (horizontal axis where it crosses the vertical axis of venous return or cardiac output) extends beyond zero to -4 mmHg (not indicated). They do not mention the sucking action of the right atrium, though.

The inescapable comparison of blood flow to the river finds its grounds in the vena cava too. Explaining how blood moves in veins, Cowan does this in a very metaphoric fashion, "The blood begins to move upward. It goes faster and faster as the large "field" coalesces into a raging central river" [160, p.19].

You can recall that in his previous comparison the narrow river meant faster flow which became "slower when it flows out into tributaries and slowest when it flows out into a wetland area" [160, p.9]. This time "field" depicts venules merging into veins where blood flows slowly which further merge into one vena cava, "a raging river." The river now is where blood moves the fastest. Nicely put but how is it possible?

As we can see from the above review, the blood flow of the venous return at the heart entrance is pulsatile, turbulent, and has high velocity, as in the aorta when it exits the heart. These features don't fit into the currently accepted "heart is an ejecting pump" theory. They indicate that the sucking function of the heart is equally strong and must be taken into consideration.

7

WHAT CAUSES HEART ATTACKS?

Coming back from our long excursion into the capillaries wonderland, we will explore an alternative explanation of heart attacks offered by Cowan. It involves the activities of the involuntary sympathetic and parasympathetic nervous systems and their effects on the heart. Our nervous system consists of the central nervous system CNS (brain and spinal cord) and peripheral nervous system called autonomic nervous system ANS, which includes nerves and ganglia (plural of ganglion, a mass of nervous tissue) carrying impulses from the CNS to organs and tissues [158, p.1565].

The autonomic nervous system has two subdivisions: sympathetic and parasympathetic branches. The sympathetic nervous system SNS, among other physiological functions, regulates heart rate, blood pressure and blood flow, and decreases insulin secretion; thus it is activated to some degree in the normal daily life [156, p.225].

Its activity greatly increases " during a stressful situation such as anger or fright, and the body responses contribute to fight or flight, ..." increasing heart rate and force of contraction [158, p.220]. Other examples of the physiological stress and increased activity of the sympathetic nervous system are excitement, exercise, injury or severe infection.

The parasympathetic nervous system PNS exerts the opposing effects: it slows down heart rate, increases secretion of insulin and digestive juices, and is sometimes regarded as "rest and digest" system [192, p.35]. Depending on certain physical and psychological tendencies, people are sympathetic or parasympathetic dominant. Such characteristics and tendencies as being tall and thin, indigestion and low appetite, high blood pressure, hyperactivity, insomnia, and irritability are features of the sympathetic dominance [192, p.36].

Personality types also play an important role in the development of heart disease. "We know that the autonomic nervous system regulates body functions by a balance between sympathetic and vagal innervation. The old distinction between "Type A" and "Type B" personalities with a physiological prevalence of one of the two systems was and still is a valid discrimination..." [193, p.84]. In this quote "vagal innervation" reflects parasympathetic activity.

The stressful way of life in the western world undermines the parasympathetic nervous system activity. "The known things that nourish our parasympathetic nervous system are contact with nature, loving relations, trust, economic security, and sex—in a sense, a whole new world" [160, p.59]. I would add, sex with a controlled ejaculation discussed in Chapter 2 of this book. Our body is designed to stay mostly in the PNS mode and shifts to the SNS mode only in emergency situations.

Following Cowan, it is an imbalance between sympathetic and parasympathetic branches of the autonomic nervous system that leads to heart disease and causes heart attacks. His focus is shifted from the coronary arteries, the darling of conventional cardiology, to the heart muscle cells and the capillaries supplying them with blood. In about three-quarters of myocardial ischemic events, the cause is not coronary artery disease but an acute reduction of the tonic parasympathetic activity [194].

The irritating factors are cigarette smoking, physical inactivity, hypertension, poor diet, exposure to environmental toxins, overindulgence in sex, and emotional stress. With this diminished parasympathetic tone, if there is a sudden surge of sympathetic activities such as physical exertion, a sleepless night, and emotional or physical trauma, then an ischemic event like angina or heart attack can occur.

What triggers the ischemic event is a sudden surge of lactic acid in the heart (myocardial) cells induced by the anaerobic metabolism of glucose. Normally, the heart uses as a fuel fatty acids, ketone bodies, lactate, glucose, and even amino acids (in starvation) to generate energy in the form of the adenosine triphosphate ATP. "Fatty acids are the predominant substrate used in the heart and generate the most ATP" [195].

Under normal conditions, the mobilization of the fuel source depends on its concentration in the blood at any particular moment. Following a carbohydrate-rich meal, the concentration of glucose and insulin increases and the heart utilizes glucose. On average, fatty acids and ketones comprise two-thirds of the heart fuel and the rest is glucose and lactate [174, p.199-200]. After an overnight fast, when glucose and insulin levels go down, the heart shifts to fatty acids and ketone bodies (produced in the liver during starvation) metabolism [196, p.125].

Whatever fuel is used by the heart, the myocardial oxygen demand for ATP production is very high. When these demands are not met, as in the case of diminished coronary blood flow due to obstructed arteries or ruptured plaque, the aerobic ATP production is shifted to anaerobic myocardial metabolism [197]. The anaerobic metabolism of glucose leads to the accumulation of lactic acid which causes a localized acidosis of the affected heart muscle.

In this acidic environment, calcium is used up and the contractile reserve of the myocardial cells is impaired [198]. The reduced ability to contract leads to localized edema and impaired muscle function in the walls of the heart. The lactic acid buildup in the cells "causes the necrosis of the tissue which we call a heart attack" [160, p.58]. This alternative explanation indicates that atherosclerosis is not the major cause of myocardial damage.

Cowan considers a proper diet as a significant means to avoid heart disease and improve heart health. "With heart disease, the most important underlying issue that we can influence with diet is the inflammation of the blood vessels" [160, p.121].

The development of atherosclerosis in coronary arteries starts early in life and to compensate for diminished blood supply, the body forms collateral blood vessels. "Gradual coronary occlusion results in the growth of coronary collaterals" [9, p.938].

Some cardiologists acknowledge the development of collateral blood vessels but do not assign a serious role to them. Little & Little describing anastomotic (between two vessels) connections, state, "...while anatomically present, they are not functionally significant and permitting collateral flow between vascular segments" [174, p.39].

However, they state, if an artery is blocked, the usually small anastomotic vessels can dilate and provide sufficient blood flow to the capillary bed in the area between functional and diseased arteries to maintain viable myocardium. "Because of the development of collateral vessels, it is not unusual to find localized severe atherosclerotic heart disease at autopsy without the presence of myocardial infarction" [174, p.40]. In other words, necrosis of the heart muscle was not the direct cause of death. Following Little & Little, collateral vessels are insignificant but somehow significant. One would see the inconsistency here, but we are all guilty of being inconsistent from time to time. At this point, Dr. Rill states: "The best collaterals in the heart provide only 20% of normal blood flow, which is enough to keep the heart muscle alive. However, at the interface between ischemic (under-perfused) and non-ischemic (normally perfused) myocardium there is a difference in myocardial electrical voltage. These particular areas are at risk for initiating arrhythmias: it is these arrhythmias that degenerate into life threatening ventricular tachycardia and ventricular fibrillation, which kill the patient."

McCance and Huether not only allocate to them an important role stating that, "...collateral circulation protects the heart" but elevate their status calling them collateral "arteries." They write,"The **collateral arteries** are really connections, or anastomoses, between two branches of the same coronary artery or connections of branches of the right coronary artery with branches of the left" [9, p. 938].

Giorgio Baroldi, MD, Ph.D., from Department of Pathological Anatomy, University of Milan, Italy and Malcolm D. Silver, MD, Ph.D., from Department of Laboratory Medicine and Pathobiology, University of Toronto, Ontario, Canada studied collaterals in great detail. They reported that in normal hearts, collateral vessels are thin-walled like capillaries but larger, "...from less than 20 to 350 μm" in diameter [142]. In diseased hearts, with blocked epicardial arteries, collateral blood vessels can reach 1-1.25 mm and are easily seen on angiography (Dr. Rill, personal communication). Notwithstanding their diameter, collaterals do not have a muscle and elastic layers as arteries do [9, p.938], thus, it is incorrect to call them "arteries."

The importance of collaterals can be appreciated if one views Dr. Knut Sroka's 5-min film in which the 90% blocked coronary artery is filled with blood before and after stenosis [199]. The heart beats normally despite a severe artery blockage and collaterals (cannot be seen in video and photographs because of their microscopic size) supply the heart muscle with blood and it functions well.

Summarizing, there are at least three hearts that govern our circulation: the heart itself, capillaries and muscles (peripheral heart). The heart must be viewed not only as an ejecting pump (arterial circulation) but also as a vacuum pump (venous return). The heart as a double-acting (ejection-suction) pump is better described as a hydraulic ram pump.

The blood flow in capillaries is controlled mostly by metabolic laws rather than by the physical fluid dynamics laws. Most heart attacks are caused by an imbalance between the sympathetic and parasympathetic nervous systems and not caused by atherosclerosis. The proposed Blood Type A1 diet, mentioned in Chapter 2, with its savory and heart-friendly lamb, eggs, butter, coconut oil, and caviar is aimed at the improvement of heart health.

8
____

THE CONCEPT OF GAIA

I f the holistic approach can be applied to the human body, mind, and spirit, which is the focal point of this book, then it possibly can be applicable to the whole Earth, our planet, as many sages, great minds, and enlightened people have suggested. Zoë Harcombe in her book, *The Obesity Epidemic: What caused it? How can we stop it?* closes her Chapter 7 with a query, "There's just one small problem to overcome–we seem to have got the idea from somewhere that nature put real fat in real food to kill us. Where did that come from?" [82, p.86]. I guess I know the answer–from Gaia.

In my understanding of the concept of Gaia, I rely on mythology, insights of sages, and scientific evidence of ecology and other related earth sciences. I have tried to expand beyond the existing Gaia hypothesis [200] to include my observations relating to the Gaia-induced longevity of some individuals rewarded with long lives for their contribution to Gaia-related global issues. Also, the Gaia perspective helps to see "the big picture," especially when we encounter hard to understand phenomena, mostly in terms of human behavior and attitudes.

In the Greek mythical tradition, the earliest deities were female Goddesses: Gaia, Pandora, Artemis, Hera, Athena, Aphrodite, and other pre-Hellenic Goddesses who preceded the Olympian Gods by

Zeus, the principal god and ruler of the other gods. Gaia was the primal Greek Goddess personifying the Earth, "...ancient Earth-Mother who brought forth the world and the human race..." [201, p.45].

The mortals envisaged a capricious Goddess "as being protective and maternal but also capable of considerable cruelty" [202, p.50]. Gaia would bless, nurture and bestow those who worshipped Her "with bountiful harvests, plentiful rainfall, and fertility, while those who turned their back on Mother Earth would be scourged by the raging elements and suffer famine and disease" [202, p.50].

The sages of the past and present spiritual teachers like Eckhart Tolle perceived the Earth as a living, conscious, and sentient entity [203, 204]. Among scientists of modern times, Vladimir Vernadsky, a Ukrainian geochemist, drafted a theory of Earth's development stating that oxygen, nitrogen, and carbon dioxide in the atmosphere were produced by biological processes.

The Gaia theory owes to James Lovelock, a British scientist who back in the 1970s formulated a hypothesis of the Earth as a living entity that sustains, nurtures and regulates life. Lovelock joined forces with Lynn Margulis, a distinguished American biologist and they assert that life on Earth determines its environment, not the other way around as orthodox scientists declare. "Life, or the biosphere, regulates or maintains the climate and the atmospheric composition at an optimum for itself" [202, p.50].

Lovelock named his hypothesis after Gaia, the Greek Mother Earth. In order for their hypothesis to be taken seriously by the scientific establishment, which would reject the notion that the Earth is a conscious and sentient being, Lovelock and Margulis, stress that Earth is "a single self-regulating, self-sustaining physiological system" [202, p.51]. As Keith Frayn's metabolic regulation [145] is concerned with the metabolism of protein, fat, carbohydrates, etc., in the human body, Earth's metabolic regulation involves global surface temperature, oceanic salinity, atmospheric oxygen, and processing of carbon dioxide.

Earth-Gaia regulates all life forms and controls their population, including the human race. At the very dawn of human civilization, when there were not many people on the face of the earth, we know of a Biblical family of Adam, Eve, and their two sons Cain and Abel. Both parents and the older son Cain tilled the soil, grew crops and made their daily bread, while Abel was in charge of the flock. Their farmer activities, such as cutting trees, making fires, polluting air with smoke and water with waste, got into Gaia's eyes and irritated her throat.

Gaia was not happy with humans who disturbed the primordial harmony that God and She created. She expressed her concerns to God who took her side and rejected Cain's agricultural food offerings such as grains subject to oxidation and rancidity and thus were of poor quality.

God welcomed Abel's natural food of scrumptious lamb, grass-fed, free of injected hormones, and replete with "heart-healthy" saturated fat derived from the grass' omega-3 by the process of bio-hydrolysis in the sheep's many stomachs, and raised on the pasture without disturbing nature, which made Cain jealous and angry. Cain could have chastised or reproached Abel but rather he, under the influence of the opiates in the bread he ate, behaved criminally and killed his brother instead [205, p.10].

Both God and Gaia, with their supernatural ESP (Extra Sensory Perception) abilities, could have foreseen and prevented a plot of a terrible crime brewing in Cain's mind. Instead, they just turned a blind eye on an anticipated murder and allowed it to happen. The first innocent soul was sacrificed and the depopulation process silently approved by God and Gaia had begun. How did Cain know how to kill? Was he influenced by Gaia? Did Gaia teach him the killing techniques?

Thus, civilization started with a conflict of interest and spread from the Garden of Eden to the whole world by population growth. More and more people disobeyed the laws of God and nature. God, overwhelmed with their sinfulness, sent a deluge to wipe out all of humanity except for Noah' family and animals. Later He sent fire from heaven and destroyed Sodom and Gomorrah, two wicked cities. But the population continued to grow and the more people there were, the more harm they did to the environment and Mother Nature.

The population reduction strategies that Gaia employed ranged from natural disasters such as volcano eruptions, earthquakes, tsunamis, hurricanes, floods, fires, etc. to epidemics such as cholera, plague, typhus, etc., to man-made disasters such as warfare and air and water pollution. Inspired by Gaia, people created more sophisticated weapons of mass destruction and successfully used them in many religious, civil, and world wars.

In their pursuit to kill each other en masse, humans discovered gunpowder, chemicals, explosives, and more recently nuclear weapons. As Tolle puts it, "Instead of killing ten or twenty people with a wooden club, one person can now kill a million just by pushing a button" [203, p.50]. Who was behind the scenes in these advancements? You guessed it, Gaia.

Gaia bestowed extended longevity to dictators responsible for millions of deaths. Among them: the Chinese communist leader, Mao Zedong (1893-1976) who was to blame for 49-78 million deaths, lived to the age of 83; Joseph Stalin (1878–1953), the Russian communist leader, caused 23 million deaths of Russians, lived to 74 (would probably have lived longer but, allegedly, was poisoned by Beria, his aide).

Yet another communist leader of Cambodia, Pol Pot (1925–1998), in his policy to create a new man responsible for the deaths of 1.7 to 2.5 million people, lived to the age of 72. The rule of the Great Leader of communist North Korea, Kim Jong-Il (1912–1994) resulted in 1.6 million deaths, lived to 82 years of age [206].

People in these communist countries lost their lives being brainwashed to believe and worship the idol of a "brighter future." As Tolle indicates, "This is a chilling example of how belief in a future heaven creates a present hell" [203, p.49]. Paradoxically, their executioners were revered as gods, living in a present paradise, and enjoying long lives. We can see that pattern everywhere, hell for the masses and heaven for Gaia's servants.

Gaia's representatives were not confined to communist countries alone. Man homicides and mass murder were always part of human history. In Europe alone, according to Tolle, "Nobody knows the exact figure because records were not kept, but it seems certain that during a three-hundred-year period between three and five million women were tortured and killed by the "Holy Inquisition," an institution founded by the Roman Catholic Church to suppress heresy" [204, p.155-6]. Tolle adds, "This surely ranks together with the Holocaust as one of the darkest chapters in human history" [204, p.156].

Another example of the Gaia's servant, the King of Belgium, Leopold II (1835–1909), who pursued the colonization of the African Congo and enslaved its people, is held accountable for 2 to 15 million deaths; he lived to the age of 73 [206]. Millions of lives were sacrificed in the World Wars.

On the wave of the industrial revolution, people began making ships, trains, planes, and cars burning coal, diesel fuel and gasoline and polluting the air tremendously. One of Gaia's beloved agents, John D. Rockefeller (1839-1937) [207], the oil magnate was instrumental in promoting the gasoline car and eliminating Nicholas Tesla's "clean-air" electric car [208]. By so doing, he forced humans to breathe exhaust fumes for more than a century, thus undermining their health and shortening their lives.

Rockefeller's another input into depopulation was making allopathic medicine a monopoly and wiping out competitive homeopathic, naturopathic, herbal, and holistic medicine [209]. That brought forth iatrogenic disease (caused by an allopathic doctor) which in 2004 claimed 740,000 deaths a year in the USA alone and became a leading cause of death [210].

For his unparalleled contribution to Her depopulation agenda, Gaia generously rewarded Rockefeller with long life—he lived to the ripe old age of 97 years and 10.5 months, 45 days shy of 98 years. Interestingly, Rockefeller himself used homeopathic medicine, as does the British Royal Family [209]. Summing up his life achievements, Rockefeller wrote a poem:

"I was early taught to work as well as play,

My life has been one long, happy holiday.

Full of work and full of play —

I dropped the worry on the way —

And God was good to me every day" [207].

And Gaia, I would add.

All these cruelties accompanying explicit disasters and wars and implicit ones such as pollution and diseases became boring and our capricious Goddess turned to a more pleasurable means—food. Everyone eats food and if that food undermines your health, it is a perfect tsunami for depopulation.

Slowly and steadily by means of the Frankenstein fats such as margarine and hydrogenated oils that are replete with *trans* fats, which are now universally acknowledged as being hazardous to health took their toll. Then Gaia initiates a war against saturated fat, which was replaced with PUFAs, carbohydrates, and *trans* fats in processed foods. This brings about an obesity epidemic, people become diabetic, suffer amputations and die by the millions prematurely from heart disease, cancer, and stroke.

We will stop here for a short while to quote Zoë Harcombe who discloses the name of an individual chosen by Gaia to create all this mess, "It became an American healthy heart strategy (launched in January 1977), on the basis of one of the most biased and fundamentally flawed studies ever to determine public health advice" [82, p.166].

Who was behind that shoddy study which gave wise to such grave consequences? His name was Dr. Ancel Keys, he was Gaia's envoy and She granted him a special award—a long life. How long did Dr. Keys live? He lived to the age of 100. Glorious!

Further, would it be possible to invent food that brings about infertility and stops people from multiplying? Yes, Gaia planted the seed of this idea into the minds of scientists and genetically modified food was born.

Do we see much sanity in the past and present self-destructive actions of humanity? If you read *The Power of Now*, by Eckhart Tolle, you are left with an impression that human race is insane," [203]. As a member of the human family, each of us, more than less, is insane too, especially in the field of nutrition.

Gary Taubes, a physicist by training, an investigative journalist, hence an outsider and critic of professional nutritionists [211], was asked after giving a lecture in a research institute by one of the faculty members: "Mr. Taubes, is it fair to say that one subtext of your talk is that you think we're all idiots?" [212, p.313].

According to Tolle's insight, the answer is a definite yes. An alternative answer, as a second opinion, comes from one doctor who replying to his patient, said, "Maybe rain, may be snow, Maybe yes, may be no, Maybe baby, I don't know." It is not that the above-mentioned faculty member and other nutritional experts are all idiots, they just do not realize that they were being used in the depopulation campaign supervised by Gaia.

By now one can be left with an impression that Gaia only punishes and kills people. It is not so. Rather, as a loving mother, She nurtures her children helping them to overcome ordeals and misfortunes. For example, She assisted them to eradicate epidemic diseases and gave people cell phones that they could communicate with each other and call to the emergency room.

Gaia granted a long life of 102 years to Fred Kummerow, a harbinger, in appreciation of his service to humanity warning it about dangers of *trans* fats. Two of Gaia's centenarian agents, Keys and Kummerow, happened to dine together in New York City. Geoffrey Cannon recalls: "Fred told me about having lunch with Ancel Keys in a fancy restaurant. They both ordered a main course of steak and eggs. Fred was surprised. Ancel Keys explained that his hypothesis was for the little people.

Later, near the end of his long life, Keys said, 'There's no connection between the cholesterol in food and cholesterol in the blood. Cholesterol in the diet doesn't matter at all unless you happen to be a chicken or a rabbit'" [213]. Does it sound like a double standard? Well, Gaia's servants including Rockefeller could get away with it, I guess.

Among centenarians whom Gaia bestowed an exceptional longevity, are George Burns, a comedian who made people laugh, thus lightening their lives, Swami Bua and Indra Devi who taught them yoga, and, of course, Jeanne Calment of France who showed how long people could live, just to mention a few.

I believe I had a touch of an encounter with Gaia during my cruise trip to Australia. Among the guests at the dinner table on the ship were Jack, 91 and his woman friend Dorris, in her early 70s. Jack, who held Ph.D. in mathematics, looked 15 years younger and his blood type was O negative.

They are quite rare and it is said that the British Royal Family members belong to O negative. In many interviews for my films there were no O negatives and I became excited at the opportunity. I asked Jack if I could videotape an interview with him. Unfortunately, Dorris who was a decision maker, declined my request on the grounds that Jack is a very private person. "Regrets, I had a few..." including this one, but what could I do?

After the cruise I stayed in Australia in four places, the last one was on the coast, in Birubi, Anna Bay, north of Sydney. The place was marvelous, with sand dunes along the 20 plus miles of beach, rocks and ocean. Each day I went for walks and videotaped rocks and waves crushing against them.

Australia is a beautiful and clean country, but I noticed some garbage between the rocks. My first thought was not to touch anything and that it is not my business to improve here anything. But one day I had an urge to collect some garbage, so I pulled a plastic bag from my pocket and started to fill it with empty cans, bottles, pieces of plastic bags, straws and broken plastic utensils.

With a bag full of my harvest, I went back to the parking area looking for a garbage can. I bumped there into Sophie, a local woman walking barefoot and we started to talk. I gave her my business card, but she couldn't read it because of her impaired sight caused by macular degeneration. Surprisingly, Sophie immediately invited me, a complete stranger, to come to her home nearby. On the way there I found out that she was 87 and her blood type was O negative. I asked her and she agreed to be interviewed. She told me her incredible story of a post-war German girl who studied in London to become a nurse, went to Fiji Islands to work in the hospital, married there a medical doctor from England, and later moved to Australia. She had a long and marvelously adventurous life.

I was utterly fascinated. What a blessing, she was four years younger than Jack, but eventually I had an interview with a blood type O negative. I had a strong feeling that Gaia granted me that interview for my having had a tiny role in the cleaning of Her environment.

Like a real rock star and a pretty woman, Gaia loves popularity and granted the Gaia theory creator, James Lovelock, 101 a long life for his unparalleled contribution to Her recognition among humans, the inhabitants of Her home [214].

CONCLUSION

The review and analysis of sex differences in life length conducted herein allows us to arrive at the following conclusions:

1. Women live five to six years longer than men. A smaller body size, less hair on the body, renewal of red blood cells through menstruation, and lower hematocrit favor women's longevity. However, the most important factor is that men when they have sex lose their semen (life force) with uncontrolled ejaculation, which women don't.

2. To make their life longer, men are advised to employ at least 14 strategies, including mastering a technique of controlled ejaculation (described in my book "Control for Life Extension. A Personalized Holistic Approach"), avoiding iatrogenic (physician caused) disease, moving south, implementing healing affirmations, being aware of a coronavirus egregore, and others.

3. The latitude of the area where people live appears to be linked to the prevalence of heart disease. In general, the closer to the equator people live, the healthier they are and the less they suffer from heart disease.

4. Conventional cardiology textbooks inadequately explain blood flow. The blood flow of the venous return at the heart entrance is pulsatile, turbulent, and has high velocity, as in the aorta when it exits

the heart. These features don't fit into the currently accepted "heart is an ejecting pump" theory. They indicate that the sucking function of the heart is equally strong. The existence of the collateral blood vessels, capillary action (a second heart), muscle contractions (a third heart) and the suction action of the heart's four chambers assisting venous blood return must be taken into account.

5. The Concept of Gaia or Mother Earth, as a conscious and sentient entity, helps us understand why humans are so sick and die prematurely. Humans exceedingly pollute and destroy Nature and Gaia punishes them to protect Herself. It seems, Her envoys, such as dictators and mass killers responsible for millions of deaths, are granted a long life.

REFERENCES

1.   https://ourworldindata.org/why-do-women-live-longer-than-men (Accessed 07/06/2019)

2. Robine J-M, Allard M. Validation of the exceptional longevity case of a 120-year-old woman. Facts and Research in Gerontology, 1995;363-7.

3. Friedman, J. Earth's Elders: The Wisdom of the World's Oldest People. Earth's Elders Foundation, Inc., 2005.

4. Shimizu K, Hires N, Ebihara Y, et al. Blood type B might imply longevity. Exp Gerontol 2004;39:1563–5.

5.   http://content.time.com/time/health/article/0,8599,1827162,00.html (Accessed 05/21/2019)

6.   https://www.dailymail.co.uk/news/article-3133888/Men-live-100-healthier-women-Male-centenarians-affected-illnesses.html (Accessed 05/21/2019)

7. Franchini M, Mingle C, Bouffant C, Rossi C, Lippi G. Genetic determinants of extreme longevity: the role of ABO blood group. Thrombosis and Haemostasis. 2016; 115.2.

8.   https://www.newsweek.com/2014/08/08/when-it-comes-long-life-there-no-gender-equality-262578.html (Accessed 05/21/2019)

9. McCance KL, Huether, SE. Pathophysiology: The Biologic Basis for Disease in Adults and Children. 4Th Ed., Mosby, Inc. St. Louis, Missouri, 2002.

10. http://lecheniebolezni.com/encreativework/teoryya-y-praktyka-profylaktyky-onkozabolevanyj (Accessed 05/21/2019)

11. https://learnodo-newtonic.com/raphael-facts (Accessed 05/21/2019)

12. Mamonov V. Control for Life Extension. A Personalized Holistic Approach. Long Life Press, 2001.

13. https://www.psychologytoday.com/intl/blog/canine-corner/201701/why-do-large-dogs-have-shorter-life-spans-small-dogs (Accessed 05/21/2019)

14. https://www.fitness19.com/body-fat-percentage-comparisons-for-men-vs-women/ (Accessed 05/21/2019)

15. Verburgh K. The Longevity Code: Secrets of Living Well for Longer from the Front Lines of Science. The Experiment, LLC. New York, 2018.

16. http://www.academia.edu/3026473/Soviet_subjectivity_Torture_for_the_sake_of_salvation (Accessed 05/21/2019)

17. Kim S-O. Penile Growth in Response to Human Chorionic Gonadotropin (hCG) Treatment in Patients with Idiopathic HypogonadotrophicHypogonadism. Chonnam Med J. 2011 Apr; 47(1): 39–42.

18. https://www.ft.com/content/70d435ca-82fb-11e5-8095-ed1a37d1e096 (Accessed 05/21/2019)

19. Fried LP, Kronmal RA et al. Risk factors for 5-year mortality in older adults. JAMA, Feb. 25, 1998, 279:8, 585-592.

20. https://www.health.harvard.edu/mens-health/marriage-and-mens-health

21. http://www.bbc.com/future/story/20151001-why-women-live-longer-than-men (Accessed 05/21/2019)

22. Kaplan SD. Retrospective cohort mortality study of Roman Catholic priests, Preventive medicine, 1988:17, 3; 335-343. (Accessed 11/29/2019)

23. Smith GD, Franke S, Yarnell J. Sex and death: are they related?

Findings from the Caerphilly cohort study BMJ 1997: 315; 1641 (Accessed 11/29/2019)

24. Persson G. Five-year mortality in a 70-year-old urban population in relation to psychiatric diagnosis, personality, sexuality and early parental death. ActaPsychiatricaScandinavica, 1981: 64, 3; 244-253 (Accessed 11/29/2019)

25. http://www.drbass.com/ (Accessed 05/21/2019)

26. Hu T, Yao L, Reynolds K, Niu T, Li S, Whelton PK, He J, Steffen LM, Bazzano LA. Adherence to low-carbohydrate and low-fat diets in relation to weight loss and cardiovascular risk factors. Obesity World, 2016: Vol. 2,1; 24-31. (Accessed 11/30/2019)

27. Ha K, Kim K, Chun OK, et al. Differential association of dietary carbohydrate intake with metabolic syndrome in the US and Korean adults: data from the 2007–2012 NHANES and KNHANES. Eur J ClinNutr. 2018: 72, 848–860 doi:10.1038/s41430-017-0031-8 (Accessed 11/30/2019)

28. Hotema H. Long Life in Florida. Health Research, 1962.

29. Willcox DC, Willcox BJ, He Q, Wang NC, and Suzuki M. They Really Are That Old: A Validation Study of Centenarian Prevalence in Okinawa. Journal of Gerontology: BIOLOGICAL SCIENCES, 2008, Vol. 63A, No. 4, 338–349. (Accessed 11/30/2019)

30. https://www.realself.com/question/liposuction-alternatives

31. https://www.cdc.gov/nchs/data/hestat/underweight_adult_07_10/underweight_adult_07_10.htm

32. Flegal KM, Graubard BI, Williamson DF, Gail MH. Causespecific excess deaths associated with underweight,overweight, and obesity. JAMA, 7 Nov, 2007; 298(17): 2028-37.

33. Kvamme JM, Olsen JA, Florholmen J, Jacobsen BK. Risk of malnutrition and health-related quality of life in community living elderly men and women: the Tromsø study. Qual Life Res., May 2011; 20(4): 575-82.

34. Arterburn DE, McDonell MB, Hedrick SC, et al. Association of Body Weight with Condition-Specific Quality of Life in Male Veterans. Amen J of Medicine. 2004;117:738–746.

35. Chapman IM. Nutritional disorders in the elderly. Med Clin North Amer 2006; 90(5): 887-907.

36. Flegal KM, Graubard BI, Williamson DF, Gail MH. Excess Deaths Associated With Underweight, Overweight, and Obesity. JAMA. 2005;293(15):1861–1867. doi: https://doi.org/10.1001/jama.293.15.1861

37. Diehr P, O'Meara ES, Fitzpatrick A, Newman AB, Kuller L, Burke G. Weight, mortality, years of healthy life, and active life expectancy in older adults. J Am Geriatr Soc. 2008;56(1):76–83. doi:10.1111/j.1532-5415.2007.01500.x

38. Uzogara SG. Underweight, the Less Discussed Type of Unhealthy Weight and Its Implications: A Review. American Journal of Food Science and Nutrition Research. Vol. 3, No. 5, 2016, pp. 126-142.

39. https://bmi-calories.com/body-fat-percentage-calculator.html

40. https://www.paleohacks.com/weightgain/how-to-increase-levels-of-subcutaneous-fat-40274

41. Jafari S, Etminan M, Aminzadeh F, Samii A. Head injury and risk of Parkinson disease: a systematic review and meta-analysis. Mov Disord. 2013; 28:1222–9. doi: 10.1002/mds.25458

42. Georgiou A, Demetriou CA, et al. Genetic and Environmental Factors Contributing to Parkinson's Disease: A Case-Control Study in the Cypriot Population. Frontiers in Neurology. 2019;10:1047 https://www.frontiersin.org/article/10.3389/fneur.2019.01047 DOI=10.3389/fneur.2019.01047.

43. https://www.scribd.com/document/348229330/The-Optimal-Diet.

44. Steele GH. The Best Way to Stay Healthy: Stay as Far Away from Doctors as You Can. Lulu.com, 2003.

45. Greger M, Stone G. How Not to Die: Discover the Foods Scientifically Proven to Prevent and Reverse Disease. Flatiron Books, 2015.

46. Lazarou J, Pomeranz BH, Corey PN. Incidence of adverse drug reactions in hospitalized patients: a meta-analysis of prospective studies. JAMA . 1998 Apr 15;279(15):1200-5.

47.   https://www.hopkinsmedicine.org/news/media/releases/
study_suggests_medical_errors_now_third_leading_cause_of_death_in
_the_us (Accessed June 10, 2019).

48. Null G, Dean C, Feldman M, Rasio D, Smith D. Death by
Medicine. Life Extension. March, 2004. www.lef.org/magazine/
mag2004/mar2004_awsi_death_01.htm

49. Null G, Dean C, Feldman M, Rosio D. Death by medicine. J
Orthomol Med. 2005;20:21–34.

50. https://insightcla.com/death-by-medicine/

51. Schwarzbein D, Deville N. The Schwarzbein Principle: The
Truth About Losing Weight, Being Healthy and Feeling Younger.
Health Communications, Inc., Deerfield Beach, FL, 1999.

52.   https://www.youtube.com/watch?v=yfXVce34A78&
feature=emb_rel_end

53. https://www.who.int/news-room/commentaries/detail/smoking-
and-covid-19 (Accessed 11/12/2020)

54.   https://en.wikipedia.org/wiki/George_Burns   (Accessed
11/12/2020)

55. Case A, Paxson CH. Sex Differences in Morbidity and Mortality. Demography, Population Association of America, 2005:42;2,189-
214.

56.   https://www.researchgate.net/publication/
5669272_Negligible_senescence_in_the_longest_living_rodent_the_na
ked_mole-rat_Insights_from_a_successfully_aging_species (Accessed
05/21/2019)

57. Bangru S, Arif W, Seimetz J, et al. Alternative splicing rewires
Hippo signaling pathway in hepatocytes to promote liver regeneration.
Nat Struct Mol Biol. 2018;25(10):928–939. doi:10.1038/s41594-018-
0129-2 (Accessed 12/29/2019)

58.   https://www.yourgenome.org/facts/why-use-the-zebrafish-in-
research (Accessed 12/29/2019)

59. Kikuchi K. Advances in understanding the mechanism of
zebrafish heart regeneration. Stem Cell Research, 2014;13, 542–555.
(Accessed 12/29/2019)

60. Major RJ, Poss KD. Zebrafish Heart Regeneration as a Model for Cardiac Tissue Repair. Drug Discov Today Dis Models. 2007;4(4):219–225. doi:10.1016/j.ddmod.2007.09.002

61. Mochii M, Taniguchi Y, Shikata I. Tail regeneration in the Xenopus tadpole. Dev Growth Differ. 2007;49(2):155–161.

62. Mescher AL, Neff AW. Limb regeneration in amphibians: immunological considerations. ScientificWorldJournal. 2006;6:1–11.

63. Endo T, et al. Brain regeneration in anuran amphibians. Dev Growth Differ. 2007;49(2):121–129.

64. González-Rosa JM, Burns CE, Burns CG. Zebrafish heart regeneration: 15 years of discoveries. Regeneration (Oxf). 2017;4(3):105–123. Published 2017 Sep 28. doi:10.1002/reg2.83

65. Kikuchi K. Advances in understanding the mechanism of zebrafish heart regeneration. Stem Cell Res. 2014 Nov;13(3 Pt B):542-55. doi: 10.1016/j.scr.2014.07.003. Epub 2014 Jul 19.

66. Spence, R., Fatema, M. K., Ellis, S., Ahmed, Z. F. & Smith C. The diet, growth and recruitment of wild zebrafish (Daniorerio) in Bangladesh. Journal of Fish Biology, 2007;71,304-309.

67. https://visiclearusa.com/b/?msclkid=b2e9eb9d0419138d13828b82f77a6db2&utm_source=bing&utm_medium=cpc&utm_campaign=VC%20-%20Search%20-%20Brand%20Name%20KWs%20-%20USA&utm_term=visiclear&utm_content=Ad%20group%201 (Accessed 02/07/2021)

68. Poss KD, Wilson LG, Keating MT. Heart regeneration in zebrafish. Science, 2002;298, 2188–2190.

69. Vivien CJ, Hudson JE, Porrello ER. Evolution, comparative biology and ontogeny of vertebrate heart regeneration. NPJ Regen Med. 2016;1:16012. Published 2016 Jul 28. doi:10.1038/npjregenmed.2016.12

70. Burda H, Šumbera R, Begall S, in Subterranean Rodents: News From Underground, S. Begall, H. Burda, C. E. Schleich, Eds. Springer, 2007, 21–33.

71. Barrionuevo WR, Fernandes MN, Rocha O. Aerobic and anaerobic metabolism for the zebrafish, Daniorerio, reared under normoxic

and hypoxic conditions and exposed to acute hypoxia during development. Braz. J. Biol. 2010;70, 425–43410.1590/S1519-69842010000200027

72. https://www.higherpeak.com/altitudechart.html

73. Baibas N, Trichopoulou A, Voridis E, et al. Residence in mountainous compared with lowland areas in relation to total and coronary mortality. A study in rural Greece. Journal of Epidemiology & Community Health. 2005;59:274-278.

74. https://www.wisegeek.com/does-altitude-affect-life-expectancy.htm

75. Darden E. The Body Fat Breakthrough: Tap the Muscle-Building Power of Negative Training and Lose Up to 30 Pounds in 30 days. Rodale, 2014.

76. https://www.huffpost.com/entry/10-toxic-people-you-should-avoid-like-the-plague_b_591344f2e4b07e366cebb80e (Accessed 02/07/2021)

77. https://www.youtube.com/watch?v=-m-rEZxw84Y&t=5s

78. https://encyclopedia2.thefreedictionary.com/Second+Signaling+System

79. https://www.youtube.com/watch?v=9TkFbM0CdJ4&t=2456s (Accessed 02/07/2021)

80. https://www.awakeningstate.com/health/thought-energy-thoughts-physical-health/

81. https://www.urigeller.com/2nd-article-on-edgar-mitchell/ (Accessed 02/07/2021)

82. https://www.lexico.com/en/definition/telekinesis

83. https://en.wikipedia.org/wiki/Psychokinesis (Accessed 02/07/2021)

84. https://en.wikipedia.org/wiki/Uri_Geller (Accessed 02/07/2021)

85. Jacić L. How a thought generates in the Human mind? 2016. https://www.researchgate.net/post/How_a_thought_generates_in_the_Human_mind/56e14a093d7f4bae2c715cc3/citation/download (Accessed 02/07/2021)

86. https://en.wikipedia.org/wiki/Swami_Vivekananda (Accessed 02/07/2021)

87. https://elesia-ebooks.e-bookshelf.de/womens-health-an-audio-recording-of-the-healing-spirit-13566816.html

88. Zaveri V. How a thought generates in the Human mind? 2016. https://www.researchgate.net/post/How-a-thought-generates-in-the-Human-mind (Accessed 02/07/2021)

89. http://www.inbooker.com/book/encyclopedia-of-healing-verbal-self-tuners-for-the-whole-family-dh088 (Accessed 02/07/2021)

90. https://nastroi-sytina.ru (Accessed 02/07/2021)

91. https://en.wikipedia.org/wiki/Autosuggestion (Accessed 02/07/2021)

92. https://en.wikipedia.org/wiki/Émile_Coué Accessed 02/07/2021)

93. https://en.wikipedia.org/wiki/Pyotr_Anokhin Accessed 02/07/2021)

94. https://настрои-сытина.рф (Sytin moods, Accessed 02/07/2021)

95. https://en.wikipedia.org/wiki/Anatoly_Kashpirovsky Accessed 02/07/2021)

96. Wolters F, Peerdeman KJ, Evers AWM. Placebo and Nocebo Effects Across Symptoms: From Pain to Fatigue, Dyspnea, Nausea, and Itch. Front Psychiatry. 2019;10:470. Published 2019 Jul 2. doi:10.3389/fpsyt.2019.00470

97. Fratello F, Curcio G, Ferrara M, Marzano C, Couyoumdjian A, Petrillo G, Bertini M, De Gennaro L. Can an inert sleeping pill affect sleep? Effects on polysomnographic, behavioral and subjective measures. Psychopharmacology (Berl). 2005 Oct;181(4):761-70. doi: 10.1007/s00213-005-0035-2. Epub 2005 Sep 29. PMID: 15986193.

98. Benedetti F, Pollo A, Lopiano L, Lanotte M, Vighetti S, Rainero I. Conscious expectation and unconscious conditioning in analgesic, motor, and hormonal placebo/nocebo responses. J Neurosci. 2003;23(10):4315-4323. doi:10.1523/JNEUROSCI.23-10-04315.2003

99. Benedetti F. Mechanisms of placebo and placebo-related effects

across diseases and treatments. Annu Rev PharmacolToxicol. 2008;48:33-60. doi: 10.1146/annurev.pharmtox.48.113006.094711. PMID: 17666008.

100. Richter M, Eck J, Straube T, Miltner WHR, Weiss T. Do words hurt? Brain activation during explicit and implicit processing of pain words. Pain, 2010;148(2):198-205

101. https://www.yahoo.com/lifestyle/the-feel-good-factor-20-ways-to-boost-your-111572466943.html Accessed 02/07/2021)

102. https://www.forbes.com/sites/nomanazish/2020/03/24/how-to-protect-your-mental-health-during-the-coronavirus-pandemic-according-to-psychologists/#728cbbd041cb Accessed 02/07/2021)

103. https://www.stressreliefcenter.com/NewCSRC/team/dr-janine-kreft/ Accessed 02/07/2021)

104. https://theosophy.wiki/en/Egregore
(Accessed 02/07/2021)

105. https://religion.wikia.org/wiki/Egregore
Accessed 02/07/2021)

106. https://en.wikipedia.org/wiki/Egregore#cite_note-8 Accessed 02/07/2021)

107. Ross CL. Energy Medicine: Current Status and Future Perspectives. Glob Adv Health Med. 2019;8: 216495611983 1221. doi:10.1177/2164956119831221

108. https://en.wikipedia.org/wiki/Mental_plane (Accessed 02/07/2021)

109. https://en.wikipedia.org/wiki/August_Kekulé#cite_note-15 (Accessed 02/07/2021)

110. Read J. From Alchemy to Chemistry. 1957. p. 179–180. (Accessed 02/07/2021)

111. https://en.wikipedia.org/wiki/Dmitri_Mendeleev (Accessed 11/12/2020)

112. https://en.wikipedia.org/wiki/Nikola_Tesla (Accessed 11/12/2020)

113. https://blog.casper.com/einsteins-theory/ (Accessed 11/13/2020)

114.   https://wiki.p2pfoundation.net/Egregores   (Accessed 02/07/2021)

115.   http://209.240.158.130/editorials/history.php   (Accessed 02/07/2021)

116. Stavish M. Egregores: The Occult Entities That Watch Over Human Destiny. Inner Traditions, 2018.

117.   https://www.watkinsmagazine.com/the-knowing-field-morphic-resonance-and-egregores

118.   http://www.jasoncolavito.com/blog/review-of-egregores-the-occult-entities-that-watch-over-human-destiny-by-mark-stavish (Accessed 02/07/2021)

119.   https://video.search.yahoo.com/yhs/search?fr=yhs-Lkry-SF01&hsimp=yhs-SF01&hspart=Lkry&p=egregore#id=11&vid=4823d288ff59b5cce733c29a5d6e72f0&action=view

120. https://www.youtube.com/watch?v=WhX94h1Tnj0

121.   https://khn.org/news/exclusive-investigation-nearly-600-and-counting-us-health-workers-have-died-of-covid-19/   Accessed 02/07/2021)

122.   https://www.earthclinic.com/latest_posts.html   (Accessed 02/07/2021)

123.   https://www.earthclinic.com/cures/coronavirus.html (Accessed 02/07/2021)

124.   https://en.newizv.ru/print?site_path=%2Fnews%2F-science%2F12-05-2020%2Fna2co3-vs-sovid-19-people-still-believe-in-fake-about-the-wonderful-properties-of-soda Accessed 02/07/2021)

125.   https://health.usnews.com/doctors/velisar-rill-169270 (Accessed 11/13/2020)

126. Ryu S, Shchukina I, et al. Ketogenesis restrains aging-induced exacerbation of COVID in a mouse model. 2020. BioRxiv preprint server.. https://www.biorxiv.org/content/10.1101/2020.09.11.294363v1

127. Mamonov V. Nutrition Mystery Solved: Why Japanese Researchers Would Never Eat Fried Food. KDP Publishing, 2020.

128. https://www.pharmacytimes.com/news/study-suggests-blood-type-a-associated-with-higher-risk-of-covid-19

129. Goldsmith JR. Vitamin D as an Immunomodulator: Risks with

Deficiencies and Benefits of Supplementation. Healthcare (Basel). 2015;3(2):219–232. doi:10.3390/healthcare3020219

130. Yang Q, Cogswell ME, Flanders WD, Hong Y, Zhang Z, et al. Trends in cardiovascular health metrics and associations with all-cause and CVD mortality among US adults. JAMA, 2012, 307:1273–1283.

131. Kheiri B, Abdalla A, Osman M, Ahmed S, Hassan M, Bachuwa G. Vitamin D deficiency and risk of cardiovascular diseases: a narrative review. Clin Hypertens. 2018 Jun 22;24:9. doi: 10.1186/s40885-018-0094-4. Erratum in: Clin Hypertens. 2018 Dec 24;24:19. PMID: 29977597; PMCID: PMC6013996.

132. Judd SE, Tanguricha V. Vitamin D deficiency and risk for cardiovascular disease. Am J Med Sci. 2009 Jul;338(1):40-4. doi: 10.1097/MAJ.0b013e3181aaee91. PMID: 19593102; PMCID: PMC2851242.

133. Wang TJ, Pencina MJ, Booth SL, et al. Vitamin D Deficiency and Risk of Cardiovascular Disease. Circulation. 2008;117:503–511 https://doi.org/10.1161/CIRCULATIONAHA.107.706127

134. Scragg R. Seasonality of cardiovascular disease mortality and the possible protective effect of ultra-violet radiation. Int J Epidemiol. 1981 Dec;10(4):337-41.

135. Petrukhin IS, Lunina EY. Cardiovascular Disease Risk Factors and Mortality in Russia: Challenges and Barriers. Public Health Reviews, Vol. 33, No 2, 436-449.

136. Menotti A, Keys A, Kromhout D, et al. Inter-cohort differences in coronary heart disease mortality in the 25-year follow-up of the seven countries study. European Journal of Epidemiology. 1993; 9(5):527–536

137. Harcombe Z. The Obesity Epidemic: What caused it? How can we stop it? Columbus Publishing Ltd., UK, 2010.

138. http://www.zoeharcombe.com/2017/08/the-seven-countries-study-part-2/ (Accessed 01/04/2020)

139. Mohammad MA, Koul S, Rylance R, et al. Association of Weather With Day-to-Day Incidence of Myocardial Infarction: A SWEDEHEART Nationwide Observational Study. JAMA Cardiol.

2018;3(11):1081–1089.   doi:https://doi.org/10.1001/jamacardio. 2018.3466 (Accessed 01/04/2020)

140.   https://www.heart.org/en/health-topics/consumer-healthcare/cold-weather-and-cardiovascular-disease   (Accessed 01/04/2020)

141.   https://nutritiondata.self.com/facts/nut-and-seed-products/3061/2 (Accessed 01/04/2020)

142. https://www.feedipedia.org/node/52 (Accessed 05/20/2019)

143. Lerch S, Ferlay A, Shingfield KJ, Martin B, Pomiès D, and Chilliard Y. Rapeseed or linseed supplements in grass-based diets: Effects on milk fatty acid composition of Holstein cows over two consecutive lactations. J Dairy Sci. 2012;95:5221–5241.

144.   https://nutritiondata.self.com/facts/finfish-and-shellfish-products/4102/2 (Accessed 05/20/2019)

145.   https://nutritiondata.self.com/facts/finfish-and-shellfish-products/4114/2 (Accessed 05/20/2019)

146.
https://www.who.int/whosis/whostat/
EN_WHS09_Table2.pdf(Accessed 01/04/2020)

147. https://www.worldatlas.com/articles/the-highest-incomes-in-the-world.html (Accessed 01/04/2020)

148.   https://www.sheffield.ac.uk/polopoly_fs/1.43991!/file/Tutorial-14-correlation.pdf (Accessed 05/20/2019)

149. https://www.worldlifeexpectancy.com/united-states-coronary-heart-disease (Accessed 01/04/2020)

150.   https://www2.bellevuecollege.edu/artshum/materials/inter/Spring04/SizeMatters/internatCardioDisSTATsp04.pdf

151. Herrera DM, Mingorance C, Rodríguez-Rodríguez R, Alvarez de Sotomayor M. Endothelial dysfunction and aging: An update. Ageing Research Reviews. April 2010;9(2):142-156.

152. Fisher MH. Death by Dentistry. Charles C. Thomas Publisher, Ltd., Springfield, Illinois, 1940.

153. Wexler L, Bergel DH, Gabe IT, Makin GS, and Mills CJ. Velocity of Blood Flow in Normal Human VenaeCavae. Circulation Research,Vol. 23, No. 3, 349-59.

154.	https://www.ncbi.nlm.nih.gov/pmc/articles/PMC3584645/ (Accessed 05/20/2019)

155. Adibhatla RM and Hatcher JF. Altered lipid metabolism in brain injury and disorders, p. 241-268. In Lipids in Health and Disease, Subcellular Biochemistry, Vol. 49, Quinn, PJ and Wang, X., Editors, Springer, 2008.

156. McCance KL and Huether SE. Pathophysiology: The Biologic Basis for Disease in Adults and Children. 8Th Ed., Elsevier, Inc. St. Louis, Missouri, 2019.

157. Esselstyn CB, Jr. Prevent and Reverse Heart Disease: The Revolutionary, Scientifically Proven, Nutrition-Based Cure. Avery, New York, 2007.

158. Taber's Cyclopedic Medical Dictionary, Venes, D., Ed., F. A. Davis Company, Philadelphia, 21 Ed., 2005.

159. Blaisdell AF. Our Bodies and How We Live. Ginn& Company, Publishers, Boston, 1902.

160. Cowan T. Human Heart, Cosmic Heart: A Doctor's Quest to Understand, Treat, and Prevent Cardiovascular Disease. Chelsea Green Publishing, White River Junction, Vermont, 2016.

161. Marinelli R, et al. The heart is not a pump: A refutation of the pressure propulsion premise of heart function. Frontier Perspectives, 1995, vol 5, no.1.

162. Webster's Deluxe Unabridged Dictionary, 2nd ed. Simon & Schuster, New York, 1979.

163. Hobbie RK, Roth BJ. Intermediate Physics for Medicine and Biology. 4Th ed. Springer, New York, 2007.

164.	https://becomingborealis.com/the-heart-is-not-a-pump/ (Accessed 05/20/2019)

165. https://en.wikipedia.org/wiki/Jean_Léonard_Marie_Poiseuille (Accessed 02/07/2021)

166.	https://www.nobelprize.org/prizes/medicine/1920/krogh/lecture/ (Accessed 02/08/2021)

167.	https://holisticprimarycare.net/topics/topics-a-g/functional-medicine/1297-blood-viscosity-the-unifying-parameter-in-cardiovascular-disease-risk.html

168. https://studopedia.su/5_10041_biofizicheskie-zakonomernosti-dvizheniya-krovi-po-sosudam.html (Accessed 05/20/2019)

169. Stein PD, Sabbah HN. Turbulent blood flow in the ascending aorta of humans with normal and diseased aortic valves. Circ Res. 1976 Jul;39(1):58-65.

170. Rhodes MJ. Introduction to Particles Technology. John Wiley & Sons, New York, 2008.

171. https://www.coheadquarters.com/PennLibr/MyPhysiology/lect5/table5.01.htm (Accessed 01/04/2020)

172. Thurston, G. B. The viscosity and viscoelasticity of blood in small diameter tubes. Microvascular Research, Volume 11, Issue 2, March 1976, Pages 133-146.

173. Marieb EN, Hoehn K. Human Anatomy & Physiology, 7th ed. Pearson Benjamin Cummings, San Francisco, 2007.

174. Little RC, Little WC. Physiology of the Heart and Circulation, 4th ed.. Year Book Medical Publishers, Inc. Chicago, London, Boca Raton, 1989.

175. Copley AL. Hemorheological aspects of the endothelium-plasma interface. Microvasc. Res. 8: 192, 1974.

176. Poisenille JLM. Recherchessur les causes du mouvement du sang dans les vaisseauxcapillaires. C. R. Acad. Sci. 1: 554, 1835.

177. Nordenström BEW. Biologically Closed Electric Circuits: Clinical, Experimental and Theoretical Evidence for an Additional Circulatory System. Nordic Medical Publications, Stockholm, Sweden, 1983.

178. Pollack GH. The Fourth Phase of Water. Ebner and Sons Publishers, Seattle, WA, 2013.

179. Bevan J. The Simon and Schuster Handbook of Anatomy and Physiology. Simon and Schuster, New York, 1983.

180. Milnor WR. Hemodynamics, 2nd Ed., Williams & Wilkins, Baltimore, 1989.

181. Jubb AP, Jubb D. Secrets of an Alkaline Body: The New

Science of Colloidal Biology. North Atlantic Books, Berkeley, CA, 2004.

182. Poole DC, et al. Skeletal muscle capillary function: Contemporary observations and novel hypotheses. Exp Physic. 2013 December ; 98(12): 1645–1658. doi:10.1113/expphysiol.2013.073874

183. https://en.wikipedia.org/wiki/Capillary_action (Accessed 01/04/2020)

184. https://www.quora.com/Doesn%E2%80%99t-blood-circulation-depend-on-capillary-action-How-else-could-a-10-oz-pump-circulate-through-100-000-miles-of-tubes (Accessed 05/20/2019)

185. Pries AR, Secomb TW. Microvascular blood viscosity in vivo and the endothelial surface layer.   Am J Physiol Heart Circ Physiol. 2005 Dec;289(6):H2657-64. Epub 2005 Jul 22.

186. http://www.rulit.me/books/endoekologiya-zdorovya-read-212312-164.html (Accessed 05/20/2019)

187. Mazumdar J, Sircar S, Saha A, and Wong K.Biofluid mechanics. World Scientific Publishing Co. Pte. Ltd., Singapore, 2016.

188. Sabbah HN, Anbe DT, Stein PD. Can the human right ventricle create a negative diastolic pressure suggestive of suction? Cathet Cardiovasc Diagn. 1981;7(3):259-67. doi: 10.1002/ccd.1810070305. PMID: 7285104.

189.   https://answers.yahoo.com/question/index?qid=20081020135547AAVgh0m (Accessed 05/20/2019)

190.   https://www.efunda.com/formulae/fluids/calc_reynolds.cfm (Accessed 05/20/2019)

191.   http://howmed.net/physiology/venous-return/ (Accessed 05/20/2019)

192. Wolcott WL, Fahey T. The Metabolic Typing Diet. New York: Doubleday, 2000.

193. Baroldi G, Silver MD. The Etiopathogenesis of Coronary Heart Disease: A Heretical Theory Based on Morphology, 2nd ed, and ©2004 Eurekah.com.

194. Sroka K. On the genesis of myocardial ischemia.   Zeitschrift-fürKardiologie. 2004, Vol 93:10, 768–783.

195. Weiss RG, Maslov M. Normal myocardial metabolism: Fueling cardiac contraction. Adv Stud Med. 2004;4(6B):S457-S463.

196. Frayn KN. Metabolic Regulation: A Human Perspective. 3 [Rd] ed. Wiley-Blackweel, 2010.

197. Katz AM . Effects of ischemia on the cardiac contractile proteins. Cardiology. 1971;56(1):276-83.

198. Martin GM, et al. Genetic determinants of human health span and life span. Progress and new opportunities.   PloS Genetics, 2007:3 1121-30.

199.   http://heartattacknew.com/heart-catheter-film/ (Accessed 05/20/2019)

200. Lovelock JE. Gaia as seen through the atmosphere. Atmospheric Environment, 1967, Volume 6, Issue 8, p.579-580.

201. Spretnak C. Lost Goddesses Of Early Greece: A Collection of Pre-Hellenic Myths. Beacon Press, Boston, 1992.

202. Roland P. New Age Living: A Guide to Principles, Practices and Beliefs. Octopus Publishing Group, Ltd., London, 2000.

203. Tolle E. The Power of Now: A Guide to Spiritual Enlightenment. New World Library, Novato, CA, 1999.

204. Tolle E. A New Earth: Awakening to Your Life's Purpose. A Plume Book, New York, 2005.

205. The New American Bible. Catholic Bible Publishers, Wichita, Kansas, 1990-1991 Edition.

206. http://www.popten.net/2010/05/top-ten-most-evil-dictators-of-all-time-in-order-of-kill-count/ (Accessed 05/22/2019)

207. https://en.wikipedia.org/wiki/John_D._Rockefeller (Accessed 05/22/2019)

208.   http://www.reformation.org/who-killed-electric-car.html (Accessed 05/22/2019)

209.   https://www.thesleuthjournal.com/western-medicine-rockefeller-medicine/ (Accessed 05/22/2019)

210. http://www.webdc.com/pdfs/deathbymedicine.pdf (Accessed 05/22/2019)

211. Taubes G. Good Calories, Bad Calories: Challenging the

Conventional Wisdom on Diet, Weight Control, and Disease. Alfred A. Knopf, New York, 2007.

212. Teicholz N. The Big Fat Surprise: Why Butter, Meat & Cheese Belong in a Healthy Diet. Simon & Schuster Paperbacks, New York, 2014.

213. Cannon G. Fred Kummerow. The man who knew about trans fats [Inspiration] World Nutrition February 2014, 5, 2, 169-173.

214. https://en.wikipedia.org/wiki/James_Lovelock (Accessed 01/05/2020)

GLOSSARY

affirmations — precisely formulated thoughts of a person about themselves, to influence the physical body and psyche, aimed to improve health, heal, and rejuvenate.

aging — the decline of any physiological, cellular or biochemical functions that occurs over time rather than from injury or disease and accompanied by a diminished probability of survival.

aldehydes — oxidation products created in the breakdown of peroxidized fats having cross-linking, mutagenic and carcinogenic properties.

amino acids — building blocks of proteins and the end products of protein digestion.

ammonia — an alkaline gas formed by decomposition of nitrogen containing substances such as proteins and amino acids. In the body, all blood gases including ammonia are in solution.

aorta — the main trunk of the arterial blood vessel system in the body, about 30 mm in diameter.

arteries — vessels carrying blood from the heart to the organs and tissues.

arteriosclerosis — a disease of the arterial blood vessels marked by thickening, hardening and loss of elasticity in the arterial walls.

arteriole — a minute artery, especially one that, at its far end, leads into the capillary.

arthritis — joint inflammation, often accompanied by pain, swelling, stiffness, and deformity.

atrium — the upper chamber of each half (right and left) of the heart.

atherosclerosis — the most common form of arteriosclerosis, marked by oxidized cholesterol-lipid-calcium deposits in the walls of arteries that may restrict blood flow and cause heart attack or stroke.

Ayurveda — an ancient Indian Traditional Medicine which takes into account body constitution determined by three metabolic principles or doshas: Vata, Pitta and Kapha. It incorporates exercise, balanced diet, detoxification, herbs, and various techniques to stimulate the circulation of prana or life force.

Blood groups or types — a genetically determined system of antigens located on the surface of red blood cells. The ABO system is of a prime importance in blood transfusions. The most common are the four blood groups: O, A, B and AB.

blood flow:

laminar — a movement of blood in parallel layers within vessel walls without disturbance.

pulsatile — a rhythmical, throbbing movement produced by the regular contractions of the heart.

turbulent — a movement of blood in disorderly currents, creating disturbances and associated with high velocity in big branching blood vessels.

capillaries — minute blood vessels, averaging 0.008 mm in diameter, that carry blood from the arterioles to the venules, supply the cells with nutrients and take away their metabolic waste.

cardiovascular disease — any disease of the heart or blood vessels, including atherosclerosis, disease affecting heart muscles (cardiomyopathy), coronary artery disease, peripheral vascular disease, and others.

centenarian — a person over the age of 100.

cholesterol — a sterol synthesized in the liver and a normal constituent of bile serving as a precursor of various steroid hormones such as sex hormones, adrenal corticoids, Vitamin D and widely distributed in body tissues. Dietary cholesterol comes from egg yolks, animal fat and organ meats, e.g. liver and kidneys.

circulation — the movement of blood through the body blood vessels.

Coronavirus Covid-19 — an infectious disease caused by the severe acute respiratory syndrome coronavirus 2 (SARS-CoV-2).

C-reactive protein — an indicator of inflammation in arteries, a predictor of heart attack risk.

diabetes — a chronic metabolic disorder marked by elevated blood glucose levels (hyperglycemia) and excessive urination. It results either from failure of the pancreas to produce insulin (type 1 diabetes) or from insulin resistance, with inadequate insulin secretion to sustain normal metabolism (type 2 diabetes).

edema (fluid retention) — a condition in which body tissues contain an excessive amount of tissue fluid.

egregore — a kind of group mind which is created when people consciously come together for a common purpose and existing on the mental plane as an autonomous entity with the ability influence people..

ejaculation — ejection of the seminal fluid from the male urethra, male orgasm.

endothelial injury — damage to the endothelial cells that line artery wall caused by oxidized cholesterol, lipid peroxidationaldehydes, e.g. MDA, HNE and HHE, smoking, diabetes, high blood pressure, elevated C-reactive protein and homocysteine, and others.

enzymes — proteins that catalyze biochemical reactions without changing their own structure.

epigenetics — changes in gene expression due to lifestyle factors such as diet and behavioral habits, and the environment.

estrogen — the female sex hormone secreted by the ovary (gland producing reproductive cells).

eunuch — a castrated man.

free radicals — highly reactive molecules containing an odd number of electrons, having an open bond and creating oxidative stress.

growth hormone — a hormone secreted by the anterior pituitary gland and regulating the cell division and protein synthesis necessary for normal growth.

HHE, 4-hydroxy-2-nonenal — reactive and cytotoxic product of peroxidation of the PUFA containing oils and fats. It was detected in inflammatory situations such as atherosclerotic lesions, in the brain of Alzheimer's and other neurophysiological disease patients.

HNE, 4-hydroxy-2-hexanal — highly reactive and toxic product of peroxidation of omega-6 containing fats and oils. HNE has been linked to such diseases as cataracts, Alzheimer's, atherosclerosis, diabetes, and cancer.

homocysteine — an amino acid which is an intermediate product in the metabolism of methionine and cysteine.

Human Chorionic Gonadotropin HCG— a hormone secreted during pregnancy by the placenta which stimulates continued production of progesterone by the ovaries and allegedly has a rejuvenating effect.

hydraulic ram — a pump that uses the water hammer effect to develop pressure that allows a portion of the input water that powers the pump to be lifted to a point higher than where the water originally started.

iatrogenic disease — a disease or symptoms induced in a patient by the treatment or comments of a physician.

interleukin — any of a class of glycoproteins (proteins that have carbohydrate groups attached to the polypeptide chain) produced by leukocytes (white blood cells) for regulating immune responses.

ketogenic diet — low carbohydrates, high fat (over 80%) diet particularly suitable for weight loss.

ketones — substances, e.g. acetone, derived from fatty acids as a source of fuel when glucose is at a short supply or there is not enough insulin in the blood.

lactic acid — substrate (substance acted upon) of glucose breakdown or synthesis (gluconeogenesis) in the liver, muscles and other tissues.

lipid peroxidation — a process under which free radicals attack and damage lipids (fats) containing double bonds, especially polyunsaturated fatty acids PUFAs.

Longevity Quotient LQ — the ratio of actual observed longevity of a specie to that predicted by their body size.

macular degeneration — an eye disease that progressively destroys the macula, the very center of the retina, impairing central vision.

metabolism — the chemical processes that occur within a living organism in order to maintain life.

metabolic syndrome — a cluster of biochemical and physiological abnormalities associated with the development of cardiovascular disease and type 2 diabetes.

metabolic waste — substances left over from metabolic processes (such as cellular respiration) which cannot be used by the organism (they are surplus or toxic), and must therefore be excreted. This includes nitrogen compounds, carbon dioxide, phosphates, sulphates, etc.

methionine — a sulfur-containing essential (must be obtained from diet) amino acid that is a constituent of most proteins.

myocardial infarction MI — another term for heart attack.

naked mole rats — nearly blind and hairless mice-like creatures living in large underground colonies in eastern Africa and marked by exceptional longevity.

obesity — the metabolic/nutritional disease marked by the unhealthy accumulation of body fat and defined as having a body mass index BMI of greater than 30 kg/m.^{2}

oxidation — a process of a substance combining with oxygen acting as a free radical and damaging it by stealing electrons.

oxytocin — a hormone secreted by the hypothalamus and stored in the pituitary gland. It causes the uterus to contract; in breastfeeding and it stimulates milk letdown.

Parasympathetic nervous system — the division of the autonomic nervous system with effects of slowing of the heart rate and increasing the secretion action of the digestive glands.

peroxidability index PI — a measure of susceptibility of fatty acids to oxidation; its value increases as the number of double bonds is increased.

Progesterone — a steroid hormone released by the **corpus luteum** that stimulates the uterus to prepare for pregnancy.

Prolactin — a hormone released from the anterior pituitary gland that stimulates milk production after childbirth.

Raphael death — as the legend goes, Raphael Santi, one of the greatest Renaissance painters died in 1520 at the age 37 due to overindulgence in sex, according to Giorgio Vasari in his book "The Lives of the Artists."

reactive oxygen species ROS — free radicals that contain oxygen and easily can react with other molecules in a cell causing damage to the cell's DNA, RNA, proteins, and can even cause cell death.

Reynolds number — value that describes the degree of turbulent flow of a liquid in a tube.

rheumatoid arthritis — a chronic inflammatory disorder that can affect joints and other body parts.

semen — the male reproductive fluid, containing spermatozoa in suspension.

stroke — a disease that affects the arteries leading to and within the brain. It occurs when a blood vessel that carries oxygen and nutrients to the brain is either blocked by a clot or bursts (ruptures).

Sympathetic nervous system — the part of the autonomic nervous system that depresses secretion, decreases the tone and contractility of smooth muscle, and increases heart rate.

testosterone — a male sex hormone that is responsible for maturation of the male sexual organs, development of sperm within the testes, sexual drive, and erections of the penis.

toxins, endogenous — toxins produced by the body as a byproduct of biochemical processes, and may accumulate in the joints or various muscle groups.

toxins, exogenous — toxins-acquired by the body through ingestion, breathing, skin contact or sometimes by injection or other medical treatment.

urea — a final product of protein metabolism in the body along with carbon dioxide; it represents a bulk of urinary nitrogen and is increased with a high protein diet.

uric acid — an end product of purine metabolism. It is a common constituent of urinary stones and gouty crystals.

vena cava — a large vein carrying deoxygenated blood into the heart. There are two in humans, the inferior vena cava (carrying blood from the lower body) and the superior vena cava (carrying blood from the head, arms, and upper body).

veins — vessels carrying deoxygenated (dark red) blood to the heart, except for the pulmonary veins, which carry oxygenated blood.

venules — tiny veins continuous with capillaries.

weight loss — a measurable decline in body weight, either intentionally or as a result of malnutrition or illness.

World Health Organization WHO — the United Nations agency concerned with international health and the eradication of disease.

worry — to experience anxiety or serious unease; allow one's mind to excessively dwell on difficulties or troubles.

yoga — a system of traditional Hindu beliefs, rituals, and activities that aims to provide spiritual enlightenment and self-knowledge. In the Western world, the term has been associated primarily with physical postures (asanas) and coordinated, diaphragmatic breathing (pranayama).

Index

ABOUT THE AUTHOR

Valery Mamonov, Ph.D., was born and educated in Russia, where he studied holistic methods and experimented with fasting, various diets, and alternative therapies for more than 20 years. He left his successful career as a consulting engineer in 1996 to concentrate full time on creating a program that would offer a new approach to health and longevity. In 2001 he published the book, "Control for Life Extension. A Personalized Holistic Approach," which was based on his research and interviews with centenarians and long-living people in the United States, Iceland, Singapore, Russia, and Japan. He is living proof of the rightness of his ideas on health: his Blood type is A (subtype A1), members of which have the shortest life expectancy of all Blood types, only 62 years. Also, he is tall, 6"2', which works against him as well: six years must be subtracted from his life expectancy because of his height. Despite of his body constitutional disadvantages, at his age of 78 he is still going strong and is free of medications. His answer is in a proper diet and a healthy lifestyle.

He had lived in Rome, Maine for 20 years and now lives in Fort Pierce, Florida.

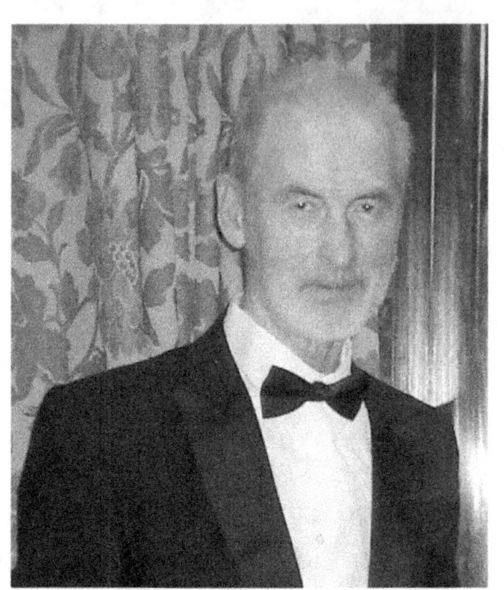

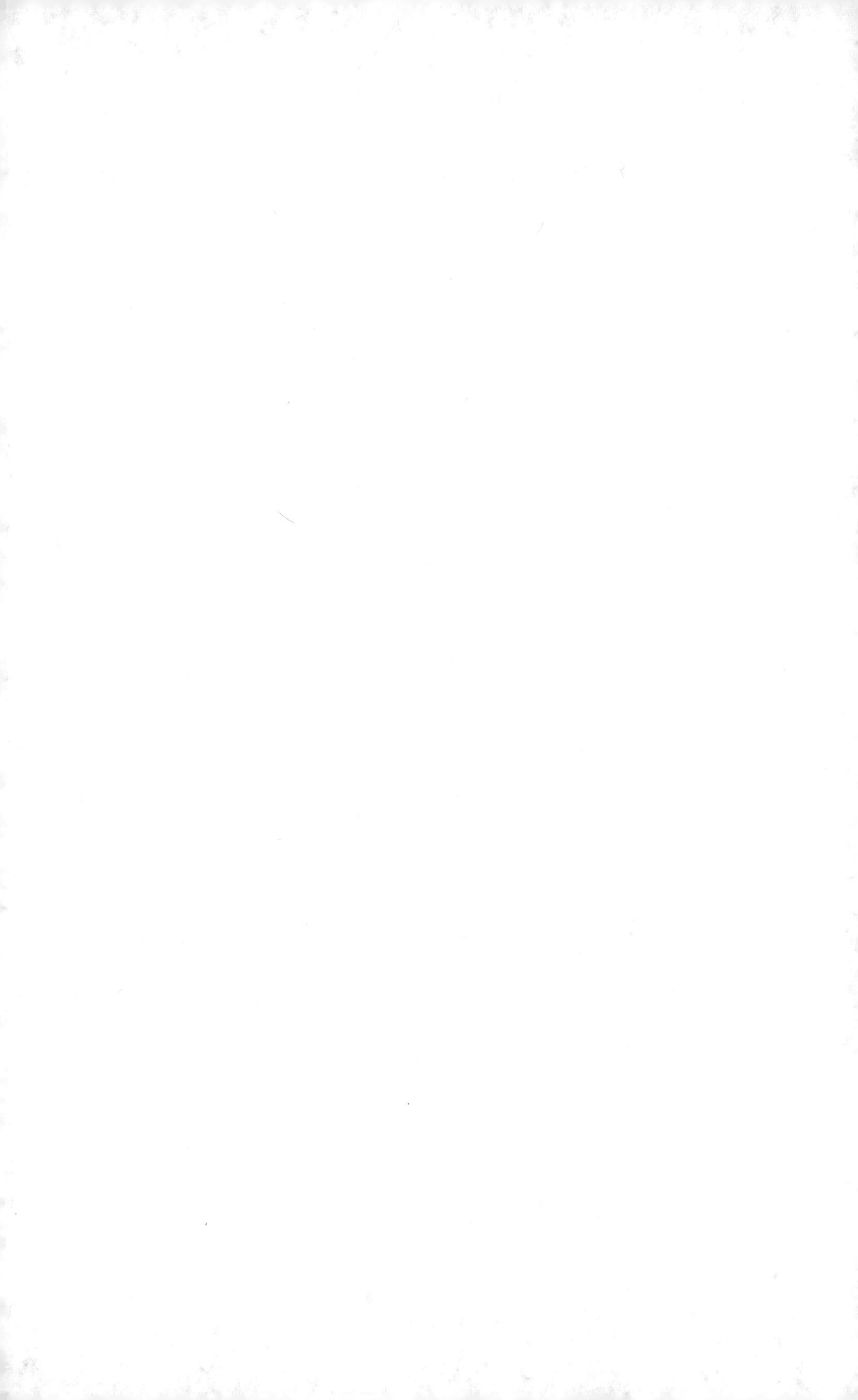